ILLUSTRATED HUMAN EMBRYOLOGY

VOLUME II

ORGANOGENESIS

by

H. TUCHMANN-DUPLESSIS, M. D., Ph. D.
Professor, University of Paris Medical School
Paris, France

P. HAEGEL, M. D.
Assistant Professor, University of Paris Medical School
Paris, France

═══

TRANSLATED BY

LUCILLE S. HURLEY, Ph. D.
Professor, University of California, Davis, California

═══

SPRINGER VERLAG
NEW YORK

CHAPMAN & HALL
LONDON

MASSON ÉDITEUR
PARIS

═══ 1982 ═══

THIRD PRINTING

I S B N   *0-387-90019-5*
3-540-90019-5
0-412-11290-6
2-225-36212-9

INTRODUCTION

EMBRYOLOGY studies the succession of transformations undergone by the fertilized egg in the formation of a new individual. Development of the embryo is directed by morphogenetic mechanisms ruled by a strict chronology. Survival of the egg, its transport in the genital tract, and the adaptation of the maternal organism to its presence are controlled by hormonal actions.

Knowledge of these subjects is proving to be increasingly important for the medical practitioner. Such information helps to explain anatomic correlations; organ relationships also illuminate the etiology of numerous pathologic conditions. Disturbances of prenatal development engender congenital malformations and constitute an important cause of perinatal mortality and postnatal morbidity.

We are grateful to numerous students and colleagues whose cooperation has aided preparation of this book.

THE AUTHORS.

TRANSLATOR'S PREFACE

Translation of this work was undertaken in order to make available in English this excellent and unusual aid for the teaching and study of mammalian, primarily human, embryology.

This book emphasizes visual presentations. It combines the use of exceptionally clear and instructive drawings with photomicrographs and concise but complete text in an exposition of the dynamic aspects of development.

Thus, the three volumes of this book will be of help in preparation and review for students, research workers, medical practitioners such as obstetricians and pediatricians, and others who are concerned with embryology. Analysis of the precise timing of various stages of human development makes it especially useful for all who are interested in the study and prevention of congenital malformations.

LUCILLE S. HURLEY.

TABLE OF CONTENTS

SKELETON

DEVELOPMENT OF MESODERM

The skeletal and muscular system develops from the third germ layer or mesoderm. It consists of:

— the axial skeleton;
— the muscular system;
— the limbs.

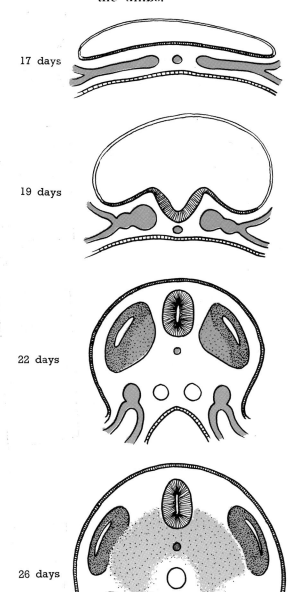

17 days

19 days

22 days

26 days

Fig. 1.

The three germ layers: in blue, the mesoderm between the ectoderm above, and the entoderm below.

The lateral mesodermal plate cleaves: appearance of the intraembryonic coelom.

Differentiation of a somite plate on each side of the neural tube.

Differentiation of the nephrogenic cord, between the somite plate and the intraembryonic coelom.

Metamerization begins about the 20-21st day, at the same time as flexion* of the embryo.

Segmentation proceeds in the caudal direction and leads to formation of 42-44 pairs of somites at the end of the 5th week.

Each somite develops a central cavity, the myocele, and on its internal side, gives rise to the sclerotome which migrates toward the notochord.

At the end of the 4th week, the sclerotome becomes polymorphous and migrates throughout the embryo. Cells derived from the sclerotome differentiate into fibroblasts, chondroblasts, or osteoblasts, according to their location.

* TRANSLATOR'S NOTE : French embryologists use the term "délimitation" to denote the overall process involving formation of the body cylinder and cephalocaudal flexion, and leading from the flat embryonic disc to assumption of the basic embryonic body form. The terms cephalocaudal flexion, or flexion, will be used here.

AND MUSCLES

SOMITE DERIVATIVES

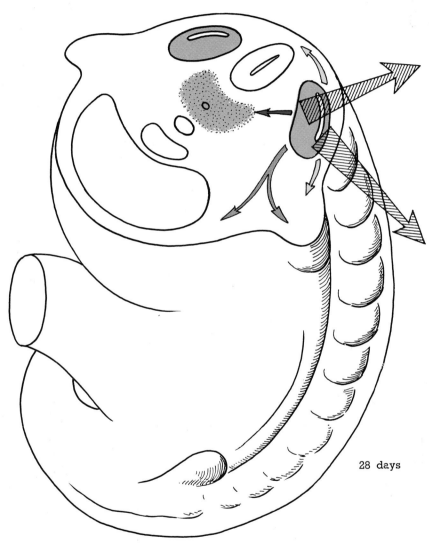

SCLEROTOME. — One part of the sclerotome groups itself around the notochord.

DERMOMYOTOME: the part of the somite which remains after migration of the sclerotome. The dermomyotome is divided into:

— **Dermatome:** mesenchyme which spreads out under the surface ectoderm to form the subcutaneous tissue.

— **Myotome:** undergoes considerable development. The cells take on a spindle-shaped appearance, and are called myoblasts.

28 days

Fig. 2. — *Somite derivatives.*

The fold which can be seen in front of the somite column is a transitory formation, Wolff's crest. The limb primordia appear at the extremities of this crest toward the end of the 4th week.

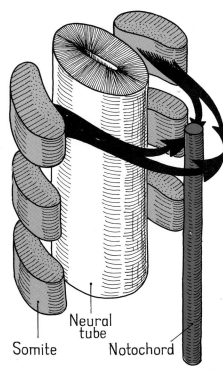

Fig. 1.

In the 4th week, the sclerotome migrates around the notochord, which thus becomes the core of a dense longitudinal column (fig. 1).

This column bears signs of its segmentary origin: blocks of sclerotome separated by less dense zones. Each level of segmentation consists of, on each side, a somite, a sclerotome mass, and the spinal nerve (fig. 2).

The caudal half of each block of sclerotome proliferates selectively, and joins the cephalic portion of the subjacent sclerotome, forming in this way the precartilaginous vertebral body (fig. 3).

Thus, the vertebral body has an intersegmental origin.

The lowest portion of the cranial half of the sclerotome block forms the *intervertebral disc* (fig. 4).

The notochord regresses at the level of the vertebral bodies, but persists and enlarges at the level of the disc, giving rise to the nucleus pulposus (fig. 5).

Definitive appearance. The paraxial musculature, derived from the somites, remains segmental.

It forms bridges from one vertebral body to another, conferring mobility and flexibility to the vertebral column (fig. 6 and 7).

The spinal nerves remain segmental and leave the vertebral column through the intervertebral foramina.

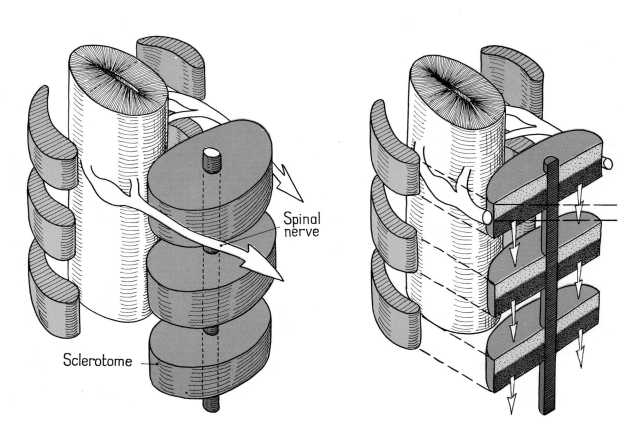

Fig. 2.

Fig. 3.

VERTEBRAL COLUMN

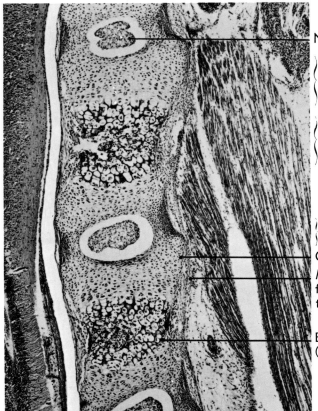

Nucleus pulposus

) Lower half of upper
(sclerotome forming
(UPPER HALF OF
) VERTEBRAL BODY

) Upper half of lower
(sclerotome forming
(LOWER HALF OF
) VERTEBRAL BODY

CARTILAGINOUS
VERTEBRAL BODY

) Area of future
(intervertebral disc

Cartilage

Muscle forming a bridge
from one vertebral body
to another.

Beginning of ossification
(example of endochondral ossification)

The posterior arches of
the vertebrae also retain
a segmental form.

Fig. 7. — *The vertebral column.*
Median sagittal section. Fetus
2 1/2 months (× 50).

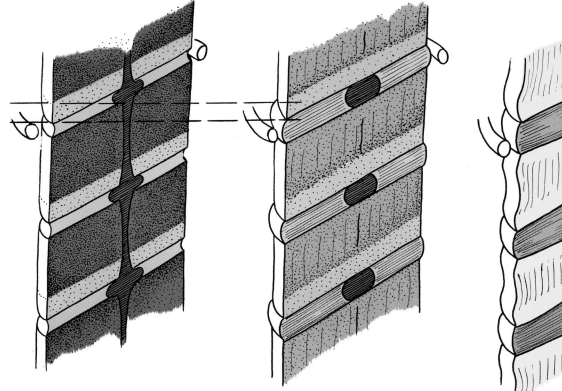

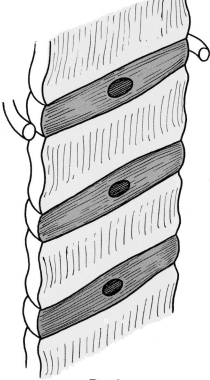

Fig. 4.

Fig. 5.

Fig. 6.

DEVELOPMENT OF MYOTOME

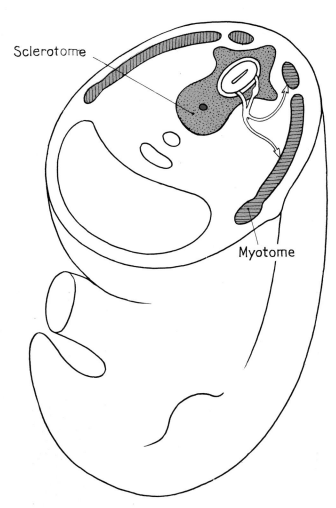

Fig. 1. — *Diagram of human embryo at 5th week.*

In the *5th week,* considerable development of the myotome takes place.

Its development is particularly clear in the thorax.

The myotome is extended in the dorso-ventral direction; it forms a small dorsal portion, *the epimere,* which will give rise to the extensor muscles of the vertebral column, and a more extensive ventral portion, *the hypomere,* which will form the lateral and ventral flexor muscles: the internal and external intercostals, and the transverse thoracic muscle.

The corresponding nerve also divides into a dorsal network destined for the epimere and a ventral network destined for the hypomere and its derivatives.

The ventral tips of the hypomeres then form buds which unite along the ventral aspect of the body, giving rise to a longitudinal muscular column, the rectus abdominus muscle.

Its initial placement is greatly modified in the abdominal wall by the meeting of muscle layers (external oblique, internal oblique, and transverse abdominus muscles).

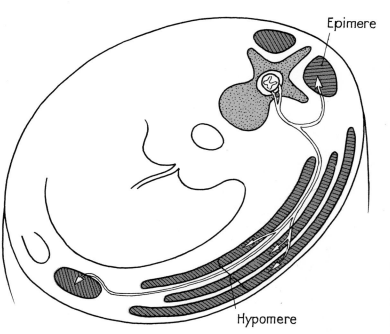

Fig. 2. — *Development of myotome.*

LIMB PRIMORDIA

The *6th week* is dominated by development of limb buds whose primordia appeared at the end of the 4th week.

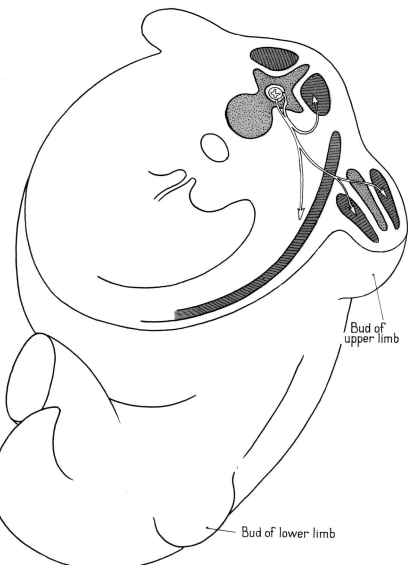

The buds are formed by a series of reciprocal inductions of mesoderm and ectoderm:

— the lateral mesoderm of the somatopleure induces a longitudinal thickening of the surface ectoderm, *the Wolffian crest,* whose middle portion disappears rapidly leaving only two nodes at the level of the future osseous girdles (see fig. 2, p. 3);

— the ectodermal nodule, on its proximal side, induces condensation of the mesoderm (sclerotome and myotome) in successive waves. Each of these in turn produces a segment of the limb, from the proximal to the distal extremity.

Bud of upper limb

Bud of lower limb

Fig. 3. — *Diagram of human embryo at 6th week.*

Innervation is brought in very early:
— for the upper limb, from the last 6 cervical and first 2 thoracic metameres;
— for the lower limb, from the last 4 lumbar and the first 3 sacral metameres.

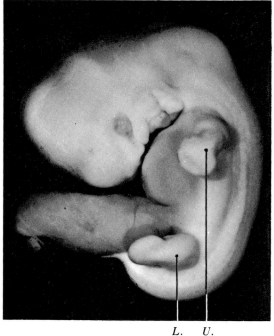

L.   U.

Fig. 4. — *Human embryo, 34 days* ($\times$ 8).
L. and *U. :* Buds of lower and upper limbs.

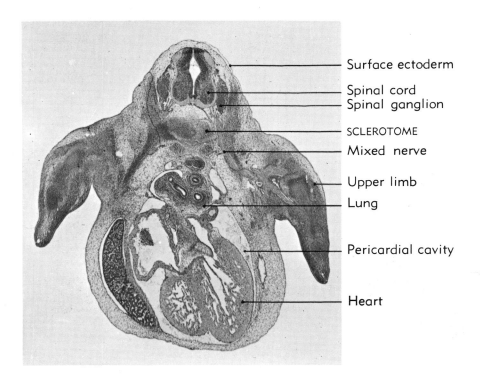

Fig. 1. — *Paddle-shaped buds of upper limbs.*
Section of thorax.
Human embryo, 34 days (× 18).

Surface ectoderm

Spinal cord
Spinal ganglion

SCLEROTOME

Mixed nerve

Upper limb

Lung

Pericardial cavity

Heart

The first primordium of the upper limb appears about the 24th day; that of the lower limb about the 26th day. The essential basic constituents can already be distinguished at 34 days.

The limb acquires its distal segment in the 7th week. After this, a groove divides the proximal segment: the limb then has its 3 definitive segments.

Development of the upper limb is more advanced than that of the lower limb (fig. 3 and 4).

Chondroblasts appear in the precartilaginous matrix which fragments to form the various skeletal parts. Between these, the first structures of the joints appear toward the 8th week (fig. 5).

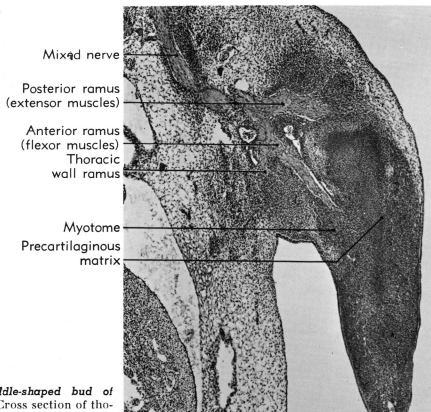

Mixed nerve

Posterior ramus
(extensor muscles)

Anterior ramus
(flexor muscles)
Thoracic
wall ramus

Myotome
Precartilaginous
matrix

Fig. 2. — *Paddle-shaped bud of upper limb.* Cross section of thorax. Human embryo, 34 days (× 50).

DEVELOPMENT

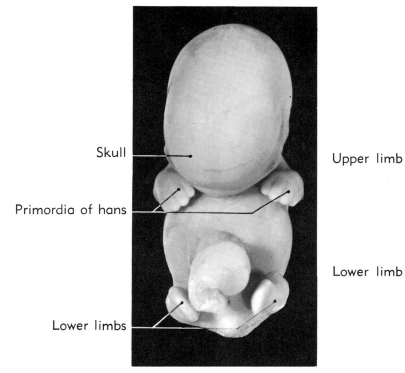

Skull

Primordia of hans

Lower limbs

Fig. 3.
7-week human embryo.
Frontal view (× 7).

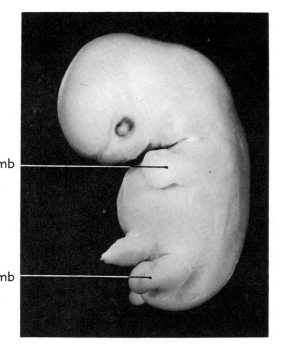

Upper limb

Lower limb

Fig. 4. — *7-week human embryo.*
Lateral view (× 7).

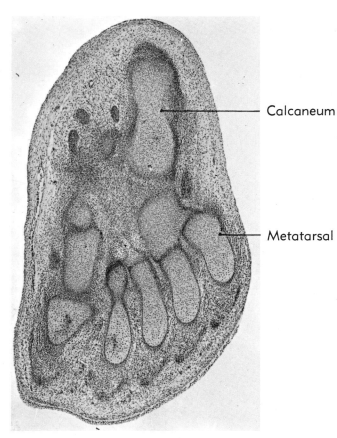

Calcaneum

Metatarsal

Fig. 5. — *Formation of joints.*
2-month fetus. Foot, longitudinal section.

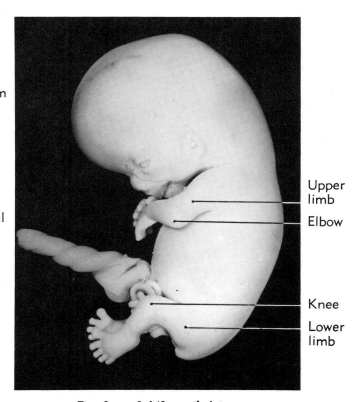

Upper limb

Elbow

Knee

Lower limb

Fig. 6. — *2 1/2-month fetus.*

LIMB ROTATION

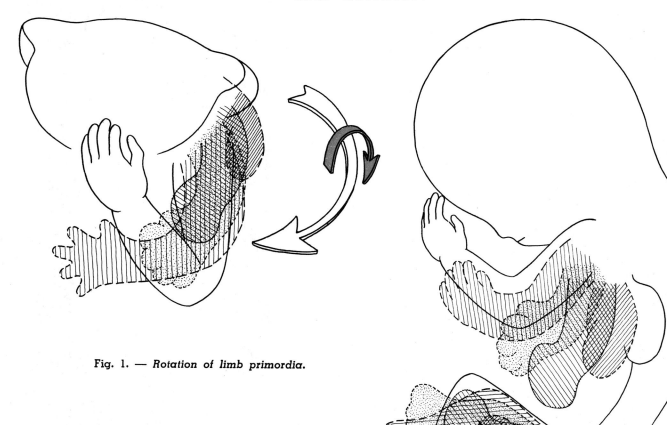

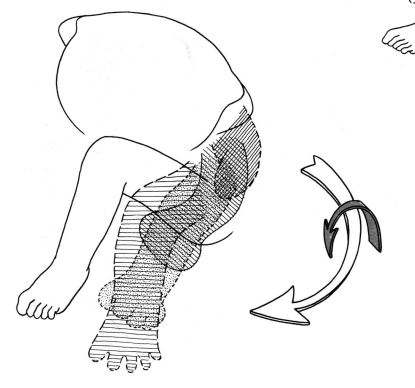

Fig. 1. — *Rotation of limb primordia.*

Fig. 2. — *Diagram of limb rotation.*

During the 8th week, while the various segments are forming, the limbs also undergo changes in orientation; the middle segment bends at an angle of 90° to the proximal segment, forming the elbow of the upper limb and the knee of the lower limb.

Finally, torsion causes the elbow to point dorsally and the knee ventrally.

LIMB MALFORMATIONS

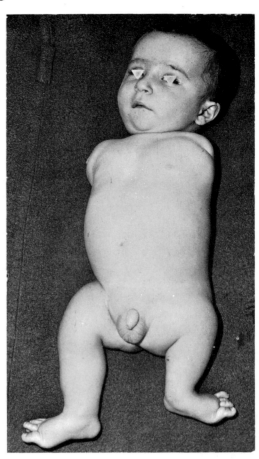

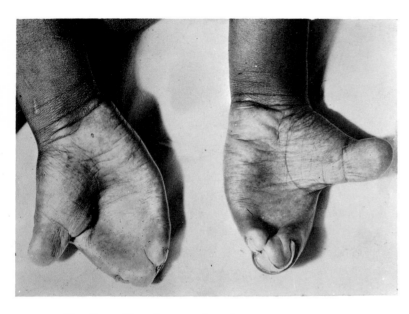

Fig. 3. — *Complete syndactyly.*
(Courtesy of Dr. B. DUHAMEL.)

Fig. 4. — *Limb malformations caused by thalidomide.* (Courtesy of Dr. DUHAMEL.)

1. The limb may be malformed as a whole: complete absence (amelia) or partial absence (ectromelia), reduction of overall size (micromelia), or reduction only in length (achondroplasia, of genetic origin).

2. Rotation of the primordia may be abnormal, leading to varying degrees of fusion (sirenomelia).

3. Malformation of only one segment of a limb may occur:

— absence of the proximal portion: phocomelia;

— anomalies of the extremities, clubbed feet or. hands, syndactyly or polydactyly (often familial);

— agenesis of the radius: absence of one of the 2 bones of the middle segment.

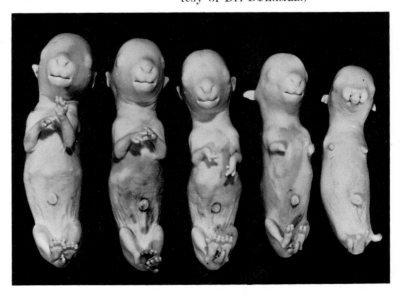

Fig. 5. — *Limb malformations produced experimentally in the rabbit.* At left, normal fetus. Almost complete array of malformations, from syndactyly to amelia.

FACIAL SWELLINGS

The face is built up from facial swellings, mesodermal masses lifting the surface ectoderm of the cranial extremity and forming the borders of a deep depression, the stomodeum, or primitive mouth.

Until the beginning of the 4th week, the stomodeum is closed posteriorly by the buccopharyngeal membrane.

There are 5 facial swellings, separated initially by grooves which are progressively filled (fig. 2).

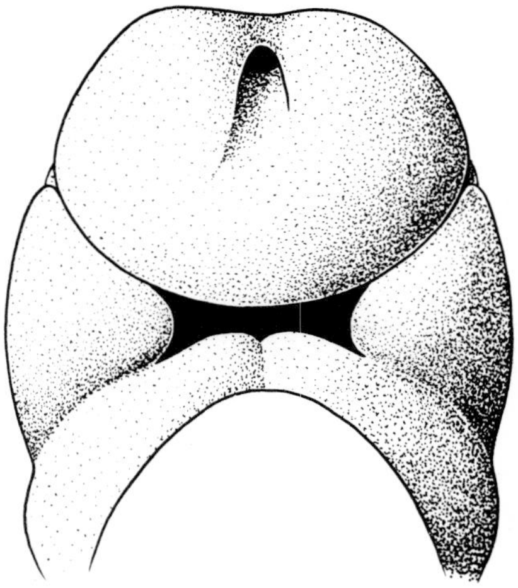

FRONTAL PROMINENCE

MAXILLARY SWELLING

MANDIBULAR SWELLING

Fig. 2. — *Face of embryo at 3-4th week.* The anterior neuropore can still be seen in the center of the frontal prominence.

The unpaired and median *frontal prominence* is the largest of the facial swellings. Determined by projection of the telencephalon, it forms the roof of the stomodeum.

The two mandibular swellings join rapidly on the midline to form the floor of the stomodeum. They represent the anterior end of the 1st branchial arch or mandibular arch.

The two maxillary swellings arise from the 1st branchial arch and form the lateral borders of the stomodeum.

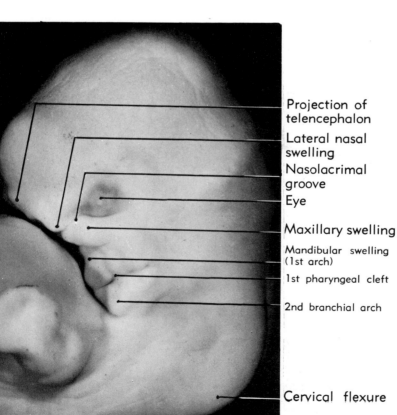

Projection of telencephalon

Lateral nasal swelling

Nasolacrimal groove

Eye

Maxillary swelling

Mandibular swelling (1st arch)

1st pharyngeal cleft

2nd branchial arch

Cervical flexure

Fig. 1. — *Profile of cephalic extremity of 34-day human embryo* ($\times$ 15).

STOMODEUM

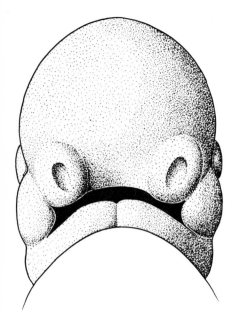

Fig. 3. — *4th-5th week:* *appearance of nasal placodes.*

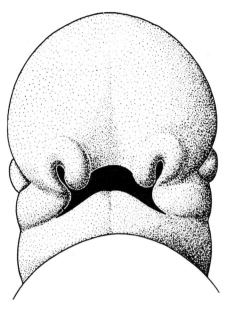

Fig. 4. — *5th-6th week:* *formation of nasal pits.*

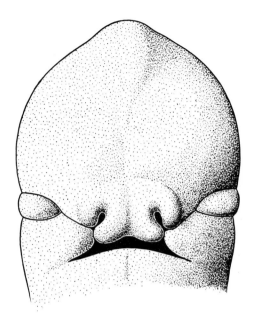

Fig. 5. — *6th-7th week:* *formation of nasal cavities.*

At the end of the 4th week, two ectodermal thickenings appear on the frontal prominence: ***the nasal placodes*** (fig. 3).

A bead of mesoderm transforms these placodes into nasal pits, which are oriented in the anterior-posterior direction at the roof of the stomodeum. The edges of the mesoderm thicken into the lateral and median nasal swellings (fig. 4).

About the 9th-10th week, the face of the fetus is almost definitively formed.

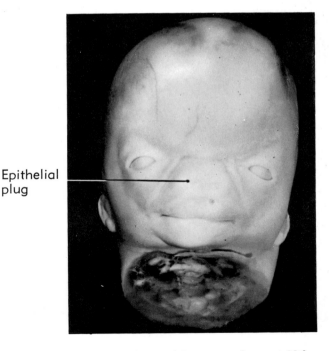

Epithelial plug

Fig. 6. — *Face of human embryo at 10th week:* the epithelial plug temporarily closes the nasal orifice (× 6).

About the 5th week, the globular process of the median nasal swelling joins the lateral nasal and maxillary swellings, closing the nasal orifice (see fig. 5, p. 13). The plane of this fusion forms the epithelial wall, which is thick and vertical ventrally, and thin and horizontal dorsally (*Hochstetter's membrane*).

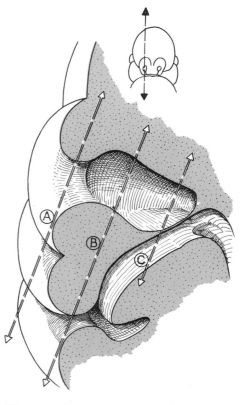

Fig. 3. — *Arrangement of 3 sections of figure 4,* opposite page. 34-day human embryo.

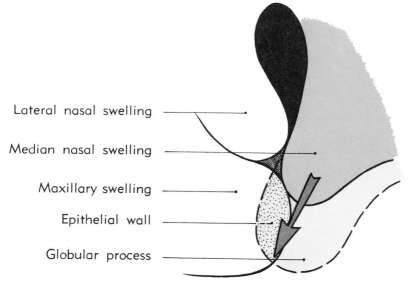

Lateral nasal swelling

Median nasal swelling

Maxillary swelling

Epithelial wall

Globular process

Fig. 1. — *Closure of the nasal pit.* Formation of the nasal orifice and the upper lip.

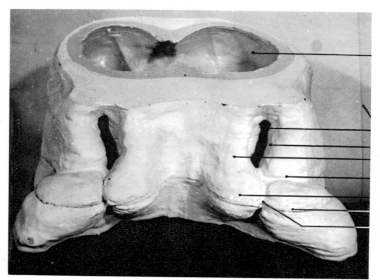

Telencephalon

Nasal fossa
Lateral nasal swelling
Median nasal swelling
Nasolacrimal groov
Globular process
Maxillary swelling
Epithetial wall

Fig. 2. — *Intermaxillary segment of 34-day human embryo.* Reconstruction.

OF NASAL FOSSAE

Fig. 4 *a* (plane A of fig. 3).

Anterior portion of nasal fossa at level of nasal orifice (× 52).

Posterior portion of telencephalon

Intermaxillary segment

Median nasal swelling

Nasal orifice

Lateral nasal swelling

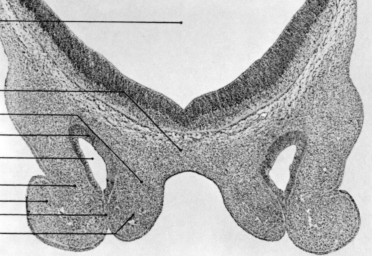

Fig. 4 *b* (plane B of fig. 3).

Middle portion : the epithelial wall results from coalescence of the median nasal swelling, the lateral nasal swelling, and the maxillary swelling (× 52).

Diencephalon

Intermaxillary segment

Median nasal swelling

Olfactory epithelium

Primitive nasal fossa

Lateral nasal swelling

Maxillary swelling

Epithelial wall

Globular process

Fig. 4 *c* (plane C of fig. 3).

Posterior portion : the epithélial wall is now represented only by the thin Hochstetter's membrane. When this opens, the primitive nasal fossa will communicate with the stomodeum (× 52).

Diencephalon

Intermaxillary segment

Primitive nasal fossa

Maxillary swelling

Median nasal swelling

Hochstetter's membrane

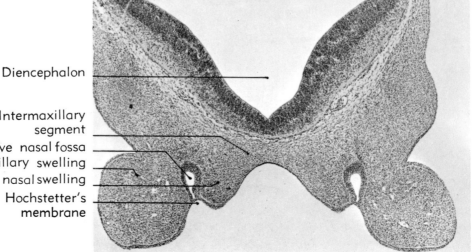

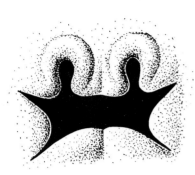
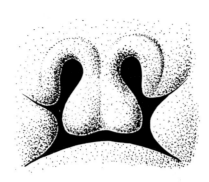
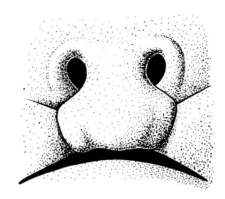

Fig. 1. — *Anterior view :* **development of the nostril.**

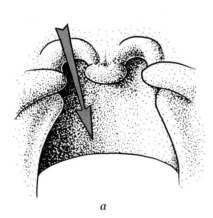
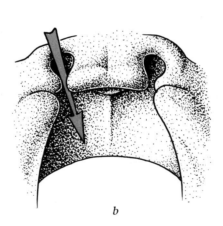
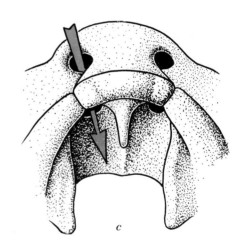

a   *b*   *c*

Fig. 2. — *Ventral view :* **the primary palate and the primitive nasal fossa.** The arrow shown through the nasal orifice marks the plane of the nasal cavity. The primary palate develops on an inferior plane.

The primary palate, separating the stomodeum from the primitive nasal fossae, is formed from the ventral side of the intermaxillary segment, limited externally by the epithelial wall. These structures form a triangular, horizontal plate with a posterior apex, the anterior palate.

The anterior palate is completely formed by the 45th day. By this stage, three formations have already appeared in the stomodeal cavity (fig. 2 C):

— a median, vertical structure, arising from the frontal prominence: *the nasal septum;*

— two lateral, horizontal structures, arising from the maxillary swellings, *the palatine shelves.*

These three plates converge and fuse on the midline, separating the definitive nasal fossae of the definitive oral cavity (fig. 2 a and 3).

OF THE PALATE

Fusion of the palatine shelves and the nasal septum begins about the 60th day. Thus *the secondary palate* is formed.

The tongue, which initially occupies the whole of the stomodeum, is pressed back in the oral cavity.

The definitive nasal fossa is formed by the primitive nasal fossa. It is completed posteriorly by the portion of the stomodeum closed off by the secondary palate. The choanae, nasopharyngeal openings, are pushed back posteriorly.

The junction between the anterior and posterior palates remains marked in the adult by the incisive foramen (fig. 2 a, F). The primary and secondary palates form the osseous palate.

The soft palate and uvula are complementary formations which appear later and form the membranous palate.

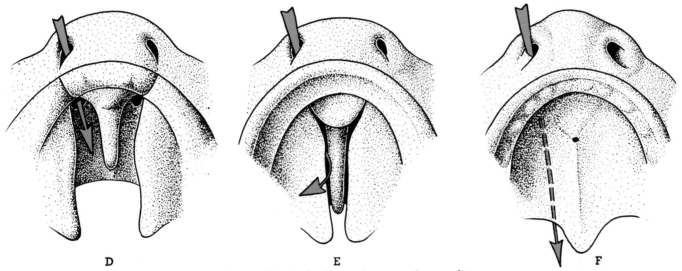

D   E   F

Fig. 2 a. — *Ventral view : the secondary palate.*

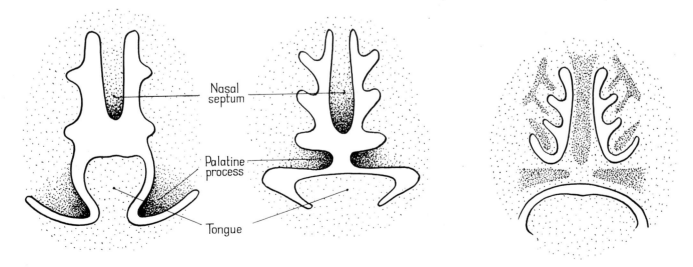

Nasal septum

Palatine process

Tongue

Fig. 3. — *Cross section : the definitive nasal fossa.*

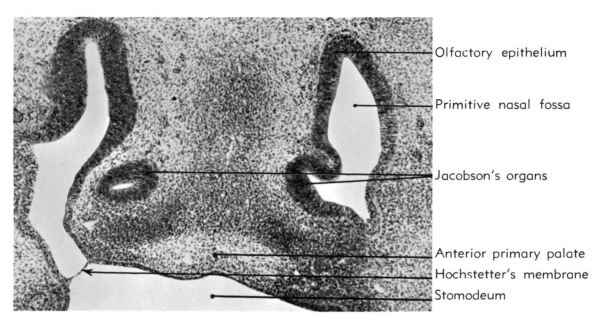

Olfactory epithelium

Primitive nasal fossa

Jacobson's organs

Anterior primary palate
Hochstetter's membrane
Stomodeum

Fig. 1. — *Primary palate.* Frontal section.
Head of rat fetus, 16 days (× 92).

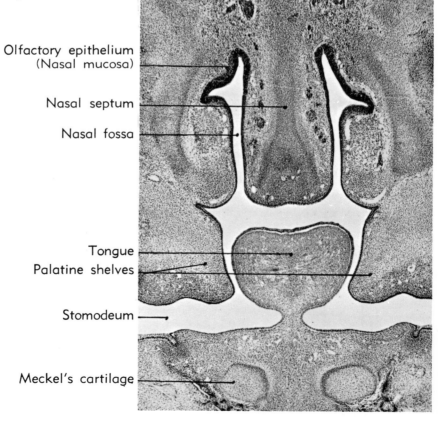

Olfactory epithelium
(Nasal mucosa)

Nasal septum

Nasal fossa

Tongue
Palatine shelves

Stomodeum

Meckel's cartilage

Fig. 2. — *Appearance of nasal septum and palatine shelves.*
Frontal section. Head of human embryo, 45 days (× 35).

The tongue is still included in the portion of the stomodeum
which will contain the definitive nasal fossae.

PALATE

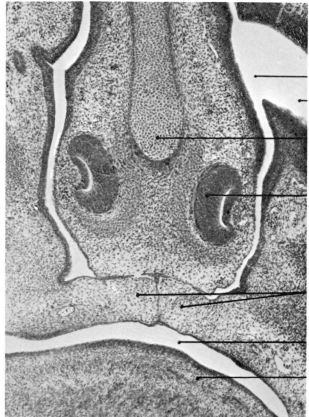

Definitive nasal fossa

Orifice of maxillary sinus

Nasal septum, with differentiation of the septal cartilage

Jacobson's organ (disappears rapidly in humans, but persists in animals)

Fused palatine shelves

Definitive oral cavity

Tongue

Fig. 3. — *Secondary palate : fusion of nasal septum and palatine shelves.* Frontal section. Head of human fetus, 60 days ($\times$ 25). Note the *line of fusion.*

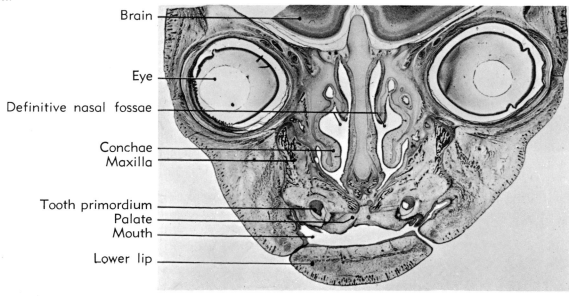

Brain

Eye

Definitive nasal fossae

Conchae
Maxilla

Tooth primordium
Palate
Mouth

Lower lip

Fig. 4. — *Definitive appearance of facial cavities.* Frontal section. Head of human fetus, 75 days ($\times$ 4.5).

Face malformations can be classified according to their date of appearance during facial development.

1. *The earliest, at the time of gastrulation* (15th-20th day): doubling of the cephalic extremity, more or less severe:

— *apodymy:* lateral doubling producing a single or double median eye;
— *rhinodymy:* doubling visible only at nose;
— *stomodymy:* doubling only at mouth.

2. *At time of formation of facial swellings* (3rd-4th week).

— **Agenesis of frontal prominence:**

— major type: *cyclopy,* incompatible with survival;
— medium type: *arhinencephaly,* agenesis of corpus callosum;
— minor type: *agenesis of nasal septum,* median fissure of nose, median cleft lip.

— **Syndrome of 1st branchial arch,** associating anomalies of the mandibular swelling and the ear: hypoplasia, median fissure. The Pierre Robin syndrome is a variation which associates micrognathy, persistent inclusion of the tongue in the nasal fossae, and cleft palate secondary to the tongue abnormality.

— **Malformations of the maxillary swelling.** These malformations are not well-defined, but are always associated through overall hypoplasia, with cleft lips and other facial fissures. Franceschetti's syndrome may be classified in this category. Here hypoplasia of the maxillary and mandibular swellings leads to unilateral facial aplasia with malformation of the ear and oblique eyelid openings slanted cranially towards the nose.

3. *At the time the facial swellings coalesce* (5th-8th week). All anomalies related to this period show up in the abnormal persistence of a fissure:

— BETWEEN THE LATERAL NASAL AND MAXILLARY SWELLINGS: *coloboma* or oblique fissure connecting the internal angle of the eye with the upper lip, without involving the nose;

— BETWEEN MAXILLARY AND MANDIBULAR SWELLINGS: *macrostomy;*

— BETWEEN THE INTERMAXILLARY SEGMENT AND OUTER SEGMENT: *harelip,* or cleft lip, with its multiple variations (frequency: 1 in 1,000 births):

— simple cleft lip which may extend to the nostril;
— cleft lip and gum, often involving the gum more seriously than the lip;

MALFORMATIONS

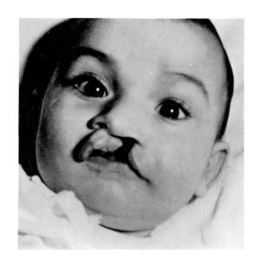

Fig. 1.
Total unilateral cleft lip.

— total cleft lip involving lip and jaw, and extending from nostril to incisive foramen;

— bilateral types, either symmetrical or asymmetrical.

— BETWEEN THE PALATINE PROCESSES: *cleft palate;* minor types are always posterior, and complete types never extend beyond the incisive foramen. (Frequency: 1 in 2,500 births).

— ASSOCIATIONS among these anomalies are multiple; only the most characteristic are cited:

— association of total unilateral cleft lip with total cleft palate, the fissure going from the lip to the uvula, and passing through the nostril;

— bilateral types are very variable for they are most often asymmetrical. The severe symmetrical form is not, however, rare: this is the classical double cleft lip and palate, total bilateral labiopalatine cleft, whose clinical appearance is striking.

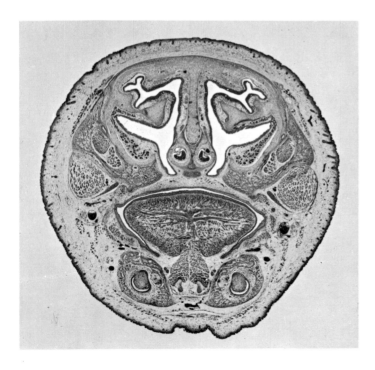

Fig. 2. — *Normal palate.*
20-day rat fetus ($\times$ 12). Frontal section of head.

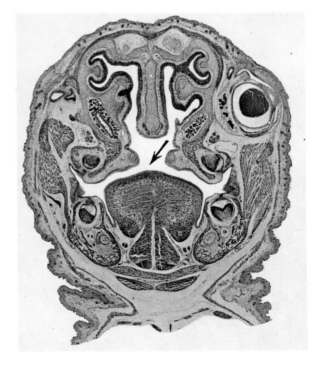

Fig. 3. — *Cleft palate.* 20-day rat fetus ($\times$ 12). The arrow marks the point where the palatine shelves have failed to fuse.

REVIEW OF EARLY DEVELOPMENT

The entoderm appears about the 8th day and rapidly forms the yolk sac. Toward the end of the first month, the process of body cylinder formation divides the yolk sac into two parts:

— one is extraembryonic (the yolk sac); it regresses early and disappears about the 3rd month;

— the other is intraembryonic (the primitive gut); it is the origin of the digestive tube and its accessory glands, the liver and pancreas.

After resorption of the buccopharyngeal membrane, the entodermal tube communicates with the exterior by the stomodeal cavity which is covered with *surface ectoderm*.

The mesoderm, formed about the 15th day during gastrulation, lines the entoderm and provides the digestive tube with its connective tissue and muscle coats and serous coverings.

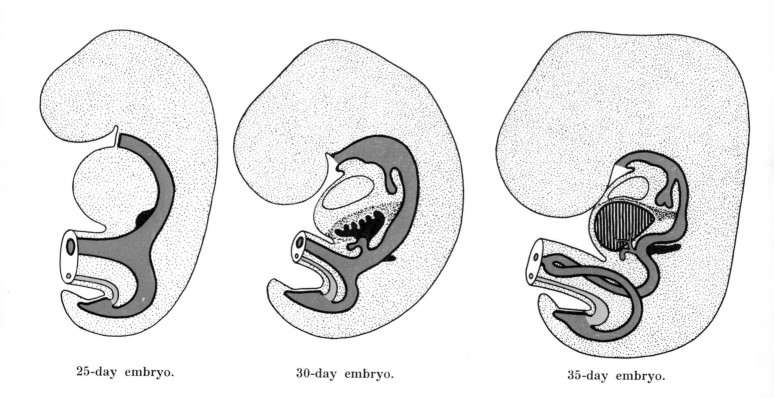

25-day embryo.   30-day embryo.   35-day embryo.

Fig. 1. — *Diagrammatic sagittal sections of human embryos.*
(At 3 stages of development of digestive system.)

SYSTEM

PRINCIPAL STAGES

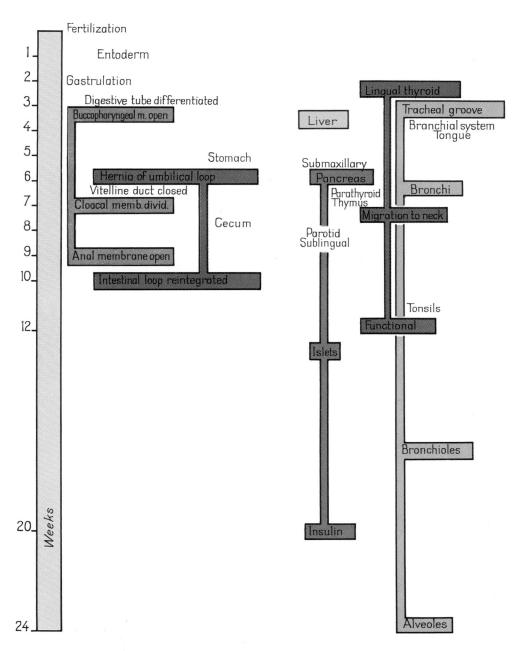

Fig. 2.

The digestive tube is initially closed by the buccopharyngeal membrane and the cloacal membrane.

— The *buccopharyngeal membrane* is resorbed at the beginning of the 4th week.
— The derivatives of the *cloacal membrane* open at the end of the 9th week.

The development of the digestive system is characterized essentially by:

— extreme complexity in its anterior pharyngeal part;
— extensive growth in length of the middle, abdominal part;
— intermingling with urogenital system in the terminal portion.

The anterior gut extends from the pharyngeal membrane to the duodenum. It is divided into a cranial segment, the pharyngeal gut, and a caudal segment composed of esophagus, stomach, and half of the duodenum.

PHARYNGEAL GUT

Modeling of the cephalic end and face of the embryo imposes a complex form on the pharyngeal segment of the digestive tube. In the three diagrams below, a cross section reveals the opened pharyngeal gut and shows its lateral walls forming **the branchial system** (fig. 1, 2, and 3).

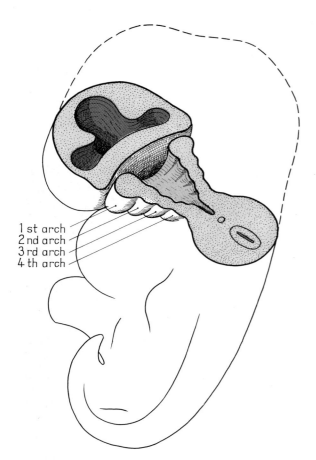

1st arch
2nd arch
3rd arch
4th arch

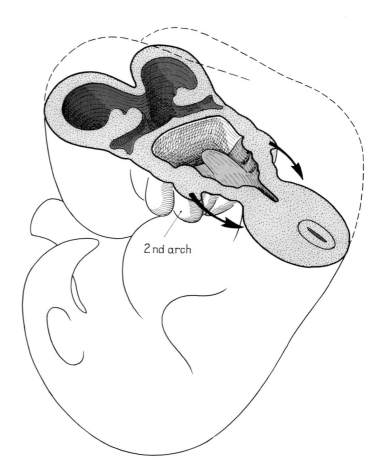

2nd arch

Fig. 1. — *Stage of about 5 mm.* The branchial system is formed, with its 4 arches, 4 pharyngeal clefts, and 5 pharyngeal pouches.

Fig. 2. — *Stage of about 8 mm.* The 2nd arch develops more rapidly than the others, and overlaps the other arches caudally. This process is accentuated by flexion of the head at this stage.

The branchial system is formed from a series of mesodermal thickenings, *the branchial arches.* These are separated by grooves visibles on the surface of the embryo as *the pharyngeal clefts,* and in the interior as *the pharyngeal pouches.*

GUT

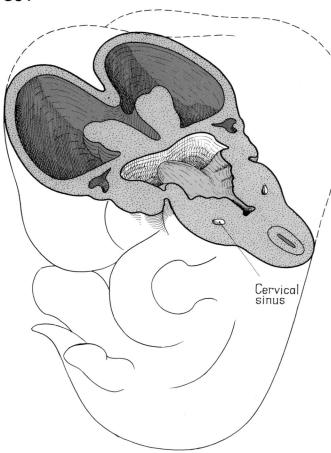

Cervical sinus

The branchial system has a transitory existence. The continuous modifications of the cephalic end of the embryo, during development of the brain, also affect the initial architecture.

— The arches give rise to skeletal structures.

— The pouches or clefts are effaced or persist only as ducts or canals. Certain of these give rise to important glandular structures.

Fig. 3. — *Stage of about 13 mm.* The 2nd arch has entirely overlapped the 3rd and 4th arches. It has closed the 2nd, 3rd, and 4th pharyngeal clefts, forming the *cervical sinus.* Only the 1st pharyngeal cleft persists, becoming the external auditory meatus.

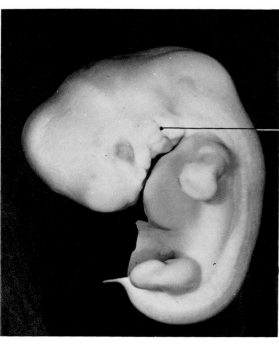

1st pharyngeal cleft

Fig. 3 a. — *Human embryo, 13 mm. 34 days. Left side.*

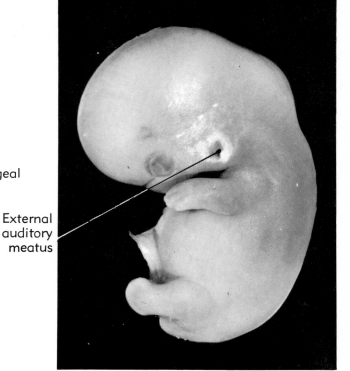

External auditory meatus

Fig. 4. — *Human embryo, 42 days. Left side.* The external auditory meatus is the only exterior evidence of the pharyngeal system.

1. Branchial or Pharyngeal Arches

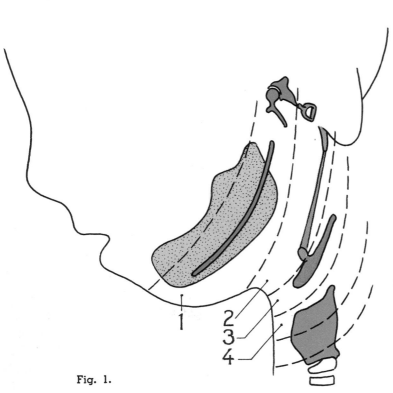

Fig. 1.

The pharyngeal arches are masses of mesoderm covered with ectoderm and lined with entoderm. Within these masses, muscular and skeletal components develop, as well as aortic arches and nerve networks.

1. *The 1st arch,* or mandibular arch, is centered on Meckel's cartilage. From its posterior portion, the malleus and incus of the middle ear arise. The mandible forms from tissue surrounding Meckel's cartilage. It is supplied by the 1st aortic arch and the inferior maxillary nerve, the mandibular branch of the trigeminal nerve (V).

2. *The 2nd arch,* or hyoid arch, is centered on Reichert's cartilage. From this arise the stapes of the middle ear, the styloid process of the temporal bone, the stylohyoid ligament and the lesser horns of the hyoid bone. It is supplied by the 2nd aortic arch and the facial nerve (VII).

3. *The 3rd arch* produces the greater horns and the body of the hyoid bone. It is supplied by the 3rd aortic arch and the glossopharyngeal nerve (IX).

4. *The 4th arch* is much less clearly differentiated. It gives rise to the cartilages of the larynx. It is supplied by the 4th aortic arch and the vagus nerve (X).

The 5th and 6th pharyngeal arches are never seen in man. Their corresponding aortic arches, however, do occur, the 6th being distinctly differentiated, while the 5th is transitory.

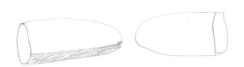

2. Pharyngeal Clefts

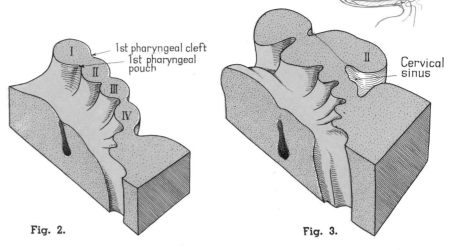

1st pharyngeal cleft
1st pharyngeal pouch

Cervical sinus

Fig. 2.

Fig. 3.

The pharyngeal clefts almost completely disappear. The 2nd, 3rd, and 4th clefts are overlapped by development of the 2nd arch. They thus form the **cervical sinus.**

This, too, disappears during extension of the cervical flexure.

The first pharyngeal cleft is the only one which persists, again only partially, to form the epithelium of the external auditory meatus.

At its external orifice, swellings arising from the mandibular and the hyoid arches participate in forming the external ear (see fig. 5, p. 29, and Vol. III).

The cervical sinus may sometimes persist in vestigial form. If it communicates only with the exterior, it forms a pharyngeal fistula, unesthetic but otherwise harmless.

However, the sinus may be open to both the exterior and the interior, forming a pharyngocutaneous fistula, and allowing saliva to run out during mastication.

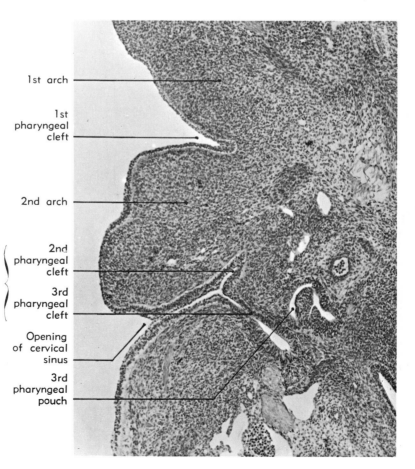

1st arch

1st pharyngeal cleft

2nd arch

2nd pharyngeal cleft

3rd pharyngeal cleft

Opening of cervical sinus

3rd pharyngeal pouch

Fig. 4. — *The cervical sinus.*
Section passing through the cervical region.
Human embryo, 34 days (× 80).

The first pharyngeal pouch elongates and appears between the internal ear and the external ear. The distal portion gives rise to the tympanic cavity, the rest to the Eustachian tube.

Fusion of the ectodermal and the entodermal layers forms the tympanic membrane or eardrum (fig. 1 and 5).

The second pharyngeal pouch elongates much less. At its extremity, the entodermal epithelium swells to form the palatine tonsil which develops *in situ* (fig. 2, 3, and 5).

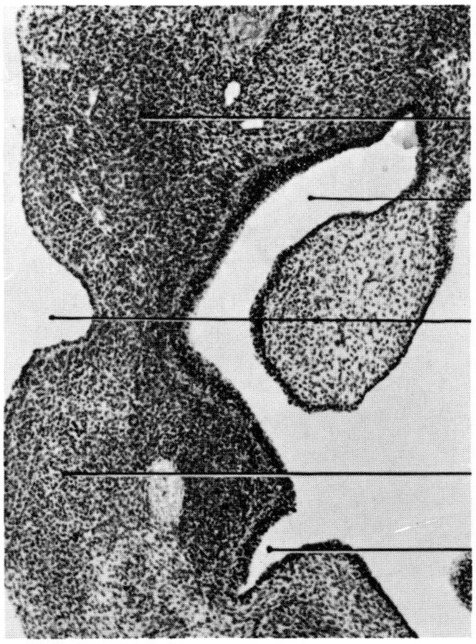

1st arch

1st PHARYNGEAL CLEFT

Tympanic membrane

1st PHARYNGEAL POUCH (distal part)

2nd arch

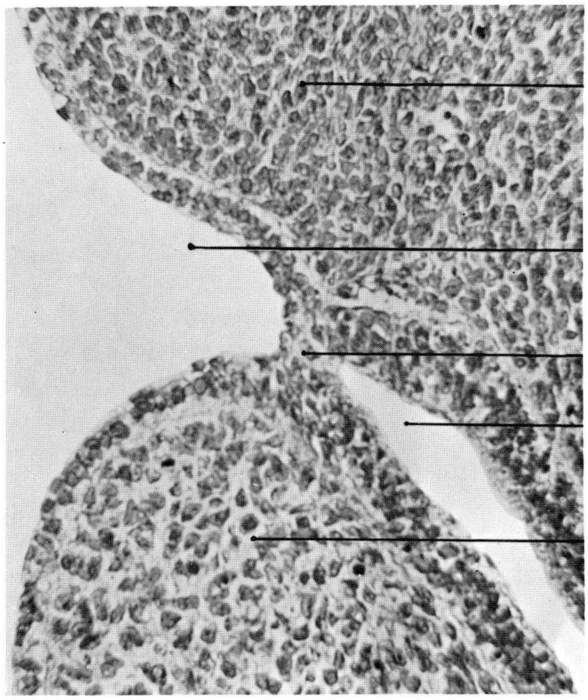

Fig. 1. — *First pharyngeal cleft and pouch.*
Section passing through cervical region. Human embryo, 34 days (× 300).

1st arch

1st PHARYNGEAL POUCH (proximal part)

1st pharyngeal cleft

2nd arch

2nd PHARYNGEAL POUCH

Fig. 2. — *First and second pharyngeal pouches.*
Human embryo, 34 days (× 65).

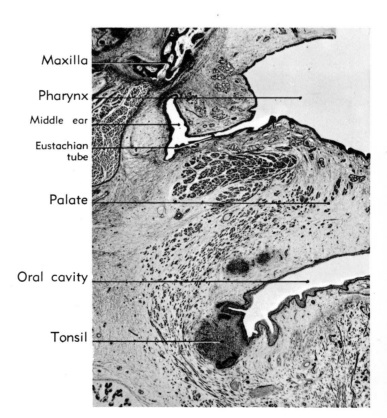

Maxilla

Pharynx

Middle ear

Eustachian tube

Palate

Oral cavity

Tonsil

Fig. 3. — *Derivatives of first and second pharyngeal pouches.*
Fetus, 3 months (× 14).

pouches

The third pharyngeal pouch provides the principal primordia of the thymus. These paired, symmetrical primordia migrate to form a single median gland located in the anterior part of the upper thoracic region. The inferior parathyroid arises from the dorsal border of this pouch and later migrates toward the posterior inferior end of the lateral lobe of the thyroid (fig. 4 and 5).

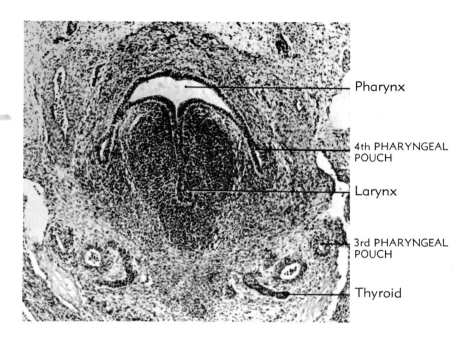

Fig. 4. — *Third and fourth pharyngeal pouches.* Section passing through cervical region. Human embryo, 34 days (× 80)

The fourth pharyngeal pouch also gives rise to a thyroid primordium. In man, however, this regresses.

The superior parathyroid arises from the dorsal border of this pouch and later reaches the superior end of the lateral thyroid lobe on its posterior side (fig. 4 and 5).

The fifth pharyngeal pouch forms the ultimobranchial body, which is thought to participate in formation of the thyroid gland (fig. 5).

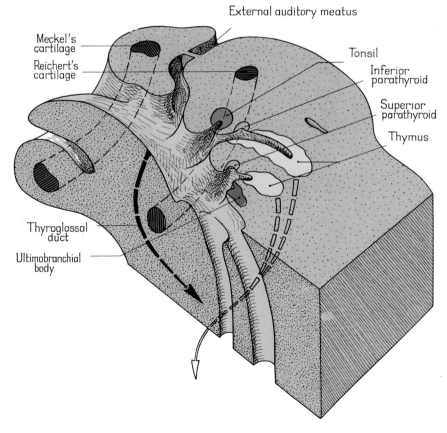

Fig. 5. — *Fate of pharyngeal pouches.*

The thyroid begins to form about the 17th day of development, from the floor of the pharyngeal gut, in the lingual primordia. It appears as a solid cellular mass between the tuberculum impar ventrally, the copula dorsally, and, laterally, the lateral lingual primordia arising from the 1st pharyngeal arch.

The glandular primordium rapidly forms an epithelial cord which penetrates the floor of the oral cavity and reaches the anterior side of the trachea. This cord hollows out into a canal whose inferior end reaches the definitive site of the gland about the 7th week. The gland then spreads out transversally into two lateral lobes. Its functional activity is apparent in the 3rd month.

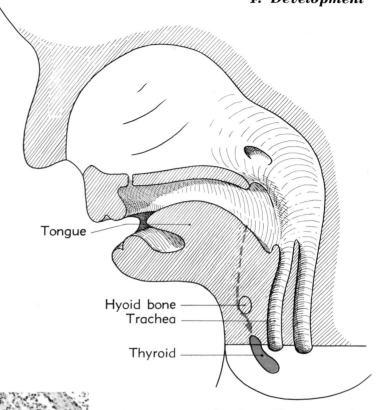

Tongue

Hyoid bone
Trachea

Thyroid

Fig. 1. — *Diagram of thyroglossal duct.*

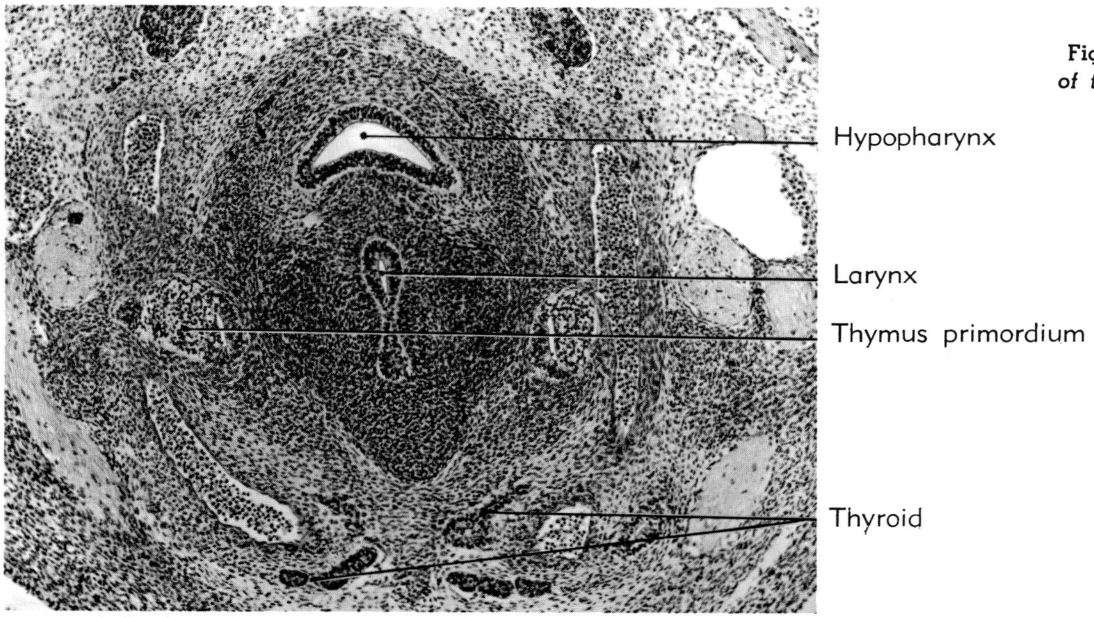

Hypopharynx

Larynx
Thymus primordium

Thyroid

Fig. 2. — *Bilateral spreading of thyroid primordium.*
Cross section of superior cervical region (× 80).
Human embryo, 34 days.

The rest of the canal forms the *thyroglossal duct* which normally regresses completely. In certain cases, however, it may persist partially as *thyroglossal cysts*. Removal of such a cyst may be necessary because of complications, but should never be done without ascertaining that there is a functioning thyroid. The cyst may be the only thyroid tissue of the body.

of the thyroid

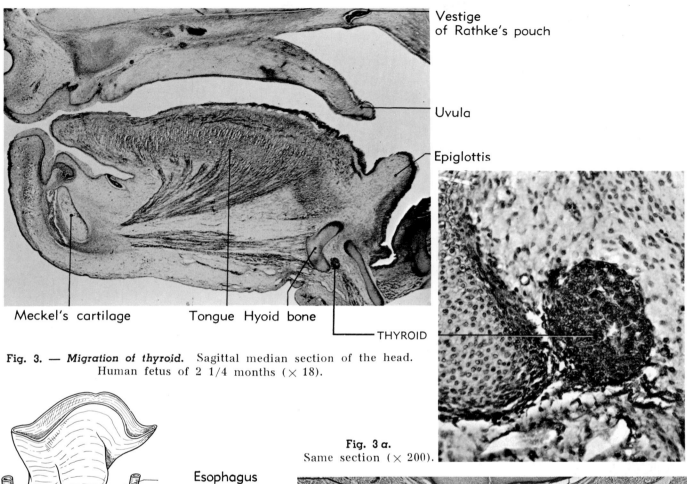

Vestige
of Rathke's pouch

Uvula

Epiglottis

Meckel's cartilage   Tongue Hyoid bone

THYROID

Fig. 3. — *Migration of thyroid.* Sagittal median section of the head.
Human fetus of 2 1/4 months (× 18).

Fig. 3 a.
Same section (× 200).

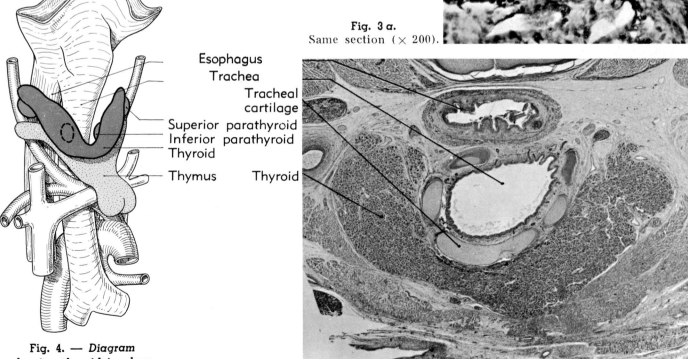

Esophagus
Trachea
Tracheal
cartilage
Superior parathyroid
Inferior parathyroid
Thyroid
Thymus   Thyroid

**Fig. 4. — *Diagram
showing thyroid in place.***

Fig. 5. — *Completely developed thyroid.*
Cross section of the cervical region (× 15).
Human fetus of 3 months.

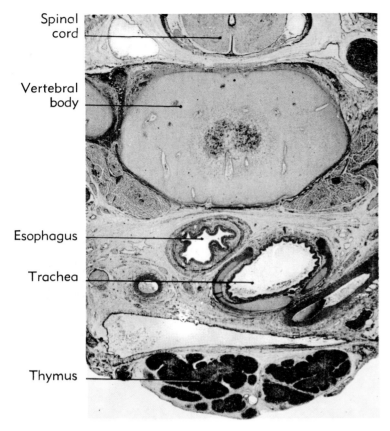

Spinal cord

Vertebral body

Esophagus

Trachea

Thymus

Fig. 1. — *Esophagus and trachea.*
Section passing through superior thoracic region.
Human fetus of 4 1/2 months (× 13).

Below the pharyngeal gut is the foregut, extending to the duodenum. Initially, it is located in the median sagittal plane and attached to the anterior and posterior abdominal walls by mesentery.

The esophagus connects the pharynx to the stomach. It remains median, and undergoes elongation due to development of the heart and retroflexion of the head. The tracheal primordium arises on its anterior side (see p. 44).

The stomach undergoes more complex changes due to growth of the hepatic primordium:

1. The posterior edge (future greater curvature) grows faster than the anterior edge (future lesser curvature) (fig. 2 *a*).

2. Rotation of 90° around its longitudinal axis displaces the greater curvature to the left, forming a peritoneal diverticulum, the future omental bursa (fig. 2 *b*).

3. Rotation along a dorsoventral axis replaces the pyloric portion to the right and upward. As a result of this rotation, the duodenum comes to lie retroperitoneally and stays there (fig. 2 *c*).

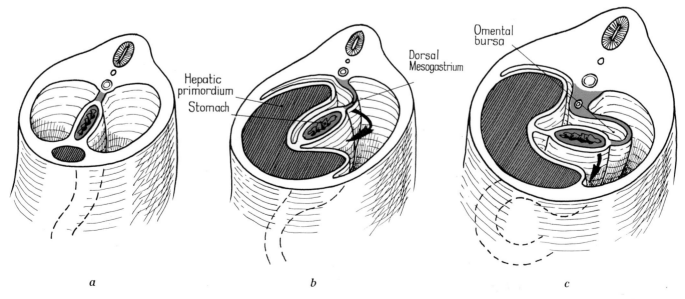

Hepatic primordium
Stomach

Dorsal Mesogastrium

Omental bursa

a   *b*   *c*

Fig. 2. — *Rotation of stomach.*

AND STOMACH

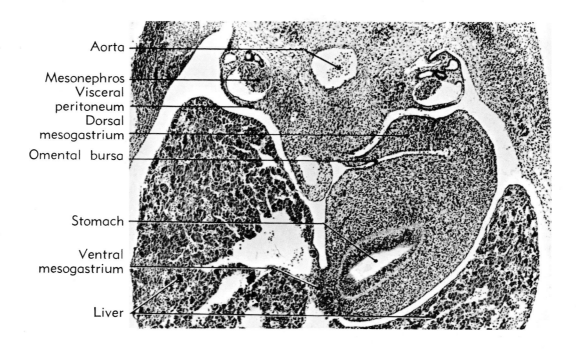

Aorta

Mesonephros
Visceral
peritoneum
Dorsal
mesogastrium
Omental bursa

Stomach

Ventral
mesogastrium

Liver

Fig. 3. — *Human embryo, 4.2 mm.* Cross section of abdomen during mesogastrium stage (× 80).

These 2 sections are at comparable levels. The one below (rat) shows a more advanced developmental stage than the one above (human).

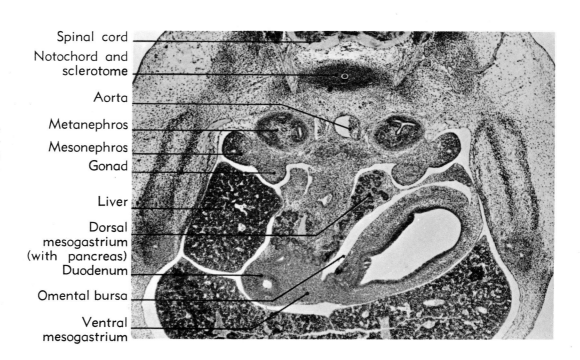

Spinal cord
Notochord and
sclerotome

Aorta

Metanephros

Mesonephros
Gonad

Liver

Dorsal
mesogastrium
(with pancreas)
Duodenum

Omental bursa

Ventral
mesogastrium

Fig. 4. — *Rat embryo, 15 days.* Cross section of abdomen at mesogastrium stage (× 40).

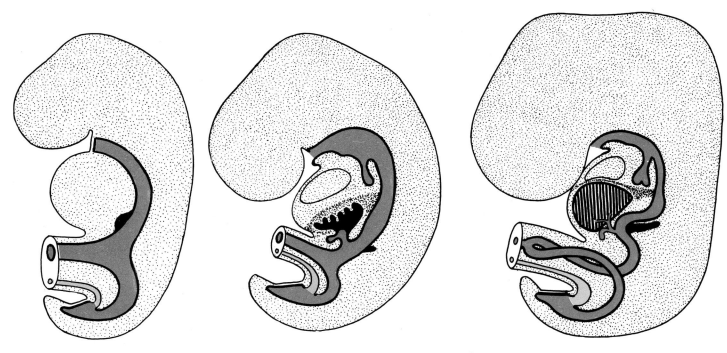

Fig. 1. — *Liver primordium at 25, 30, and 35 days.*

The liver primordium appears about the 3rd week, as a ventral thickening of the entoderm at the distal end of the foregut (future duodenum).

The major portion of this primordium produces the hepatic parenchyma and the main bile duct. A secondary, caudal, proliferation will become the gall bladder and the cystic duct (fig. 1 and 3 *a*).

The hepatic primordium is formed of cellular cords which colonize the ventral mesogastrium (septum transversum). These cords bring about fragmentation of the veins supplying the liver into a sinusoid network (vitelline and umbilical veins, see p. 130).

About the 10th week, the liver makes up approximately 1/10 of the total fetal body weight. Between the 2nd and 7th months, the fetal liver has an important role in hematopoiesis.

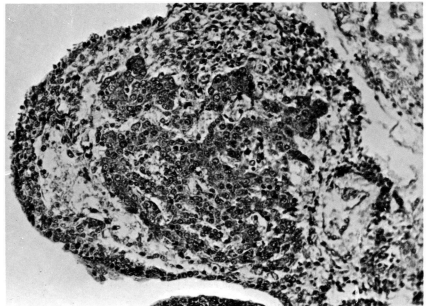

Fig. 2. — *Liver cords in the septum transversum.* Human embryo. 4th week (× 410).

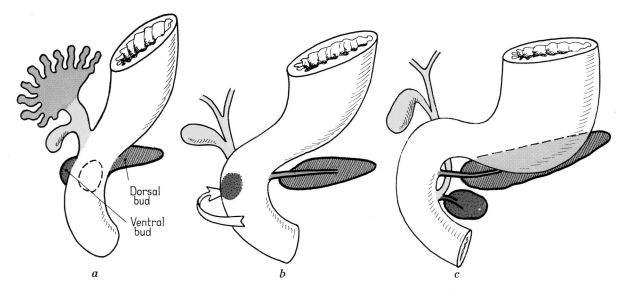

Fig. 3 *a, b, c,* and *d.* — *Pancreatic primordia.*

The pancreas appears in the 5th week, from a dorsal bud above the hepatic diverticulum, and from a ventral bud in the angle below the hepatic rudiment.

The dorsal bud gives rise to the upper half of the head of the pancreas, the isthmus, the body, and the tail; its excretory duct is the accessory pancreatic duct of Santorini.

The ventral bud migrates with the lower end of the common bile duct and fuses with the dorsal bud in the dorsal mesogastrium. It forms the lower half of the head of the pancreas. Its excretory duct collects the secretion of the major part of the dorsal portion; this is the duct of Wirsung, or combined pancreatic duct.

The common bile duct and duct of Wirsung open into Vater's ampulla in the 2nd part of the duodenum, either together or separately, with the common bile duct above the duct of Wirsung.

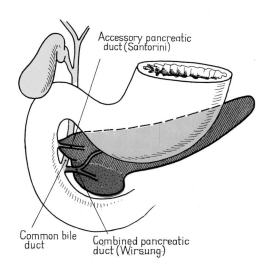

Fig. 3 d.

Fig. 4. — *Longitudinal section of duodenal-pancreatic block.* Human fetus, 4 1/2 months ($\times$ 6).

D_1 = 1st part of duodenum; D_2 = 2nd part of duodenum.

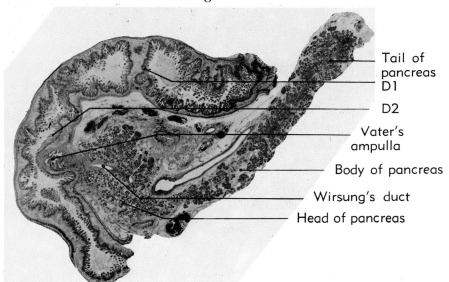

PRIMITIVE GUT-LOOP

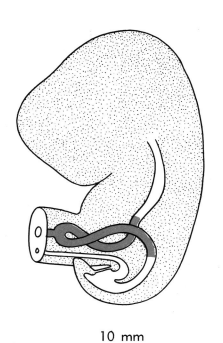 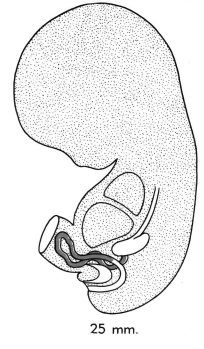 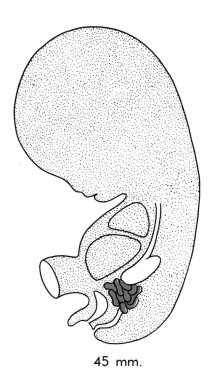

10 mm   25 mm.   45 mm.

Fig. 1.

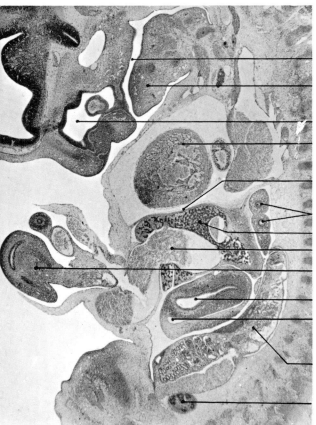

Stomodeum

Tongue

Nasal fossa

Heart

Diaphragm

Lung

Liver

Umbilical vein

Physiological hernia

Stomach

Omental bursa

Mesonephros

Metanephros

The gut-loop, or midgut begins immediately caudal to the entrance of the bile duct into the duodenum and ends at the beginning of the last third of the transverse colon.

The principal characteristics of its development is its extraordinary growth in length.

The midgut develops almost entirely outside the abdominal cavity, in the extra-embryonic coelom of the umbilical cord. This is the *physiological hernia* seen from the 6th to the 10th weeks.

In the 10th week, the gut returns to the abdominal cavity, requiring an adaptation which completely changes its original orientation (fig. 1).

Fig. 2. — *Physiological hernia, containing intestinal loops* in coelom of umbilical cord.

Sagittal median section. Rabbit fetus, 14 days ($\times$ 18).

ROTATION OF INTESTINAL LOOP

The intestinal mass undergoes a complex counterclockwise rotation (seen from anterior). The theoretical axis is represented by the superior mesenteric artery and the vitelline duct.

Fig. 3. — *Primitive gut loop,* in sagittal plane, around axis of superior mesenteric artery. From this artery there arise the colic branches for the caudal limb of primitive gut loop, and the jejunoileal branches for the cranial limb of primitive gut loop. At its apex, the vitelline duct.

Fig. 5. — *Rotation through 180° and swing towards frontal plane.* The colic branches are now above the jejunoileal branches. The caecum is under the liver. The vitelline duct regresses. The cranial limb of the gut loop forms the jejunoileal loops. The caudal limb forms the end of the ileum and part of the colon.

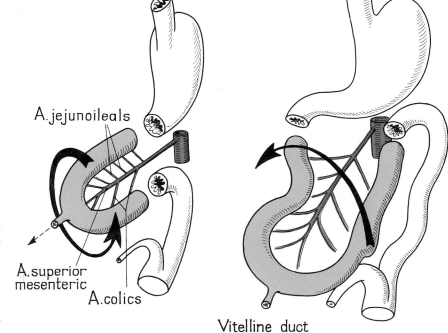

Fig. 3.

Fig. 4.

Fig. 4. — *Rotation through 90°.* The colic branches are at left, the ileal branches at right. At the same time, the stomach moves into the frontal plane. The caecal bud appears on the caudal limb of the primitive gut loop.

Fig. 6. — *Definitive arrangement.* Rotation is over. The caecum descends into the right iliac fossa by simple elongation. The appendix is a vestige of the incomplete development of the caecum. The duodenum is now completely fixed in position.

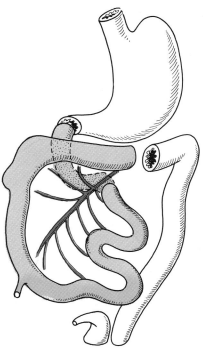

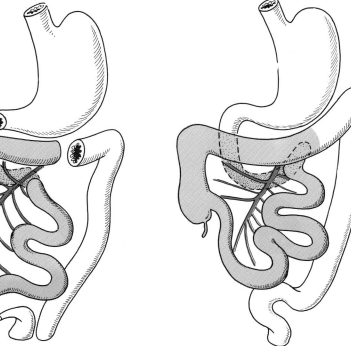

Fig. 5.

Fig. 6.

Intestinal malformations may result from abnormal development of the digestive tube itself, from abnormalities in its location and arrangement, or from defective development of the neighboring organs. Several causes may often be interconnected. Their major clinical manifestation is a syndrome of neonatal intestinal obstruction.

I. — ANOMALIES OF DEVELOPMENT

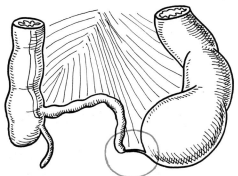

Fig. 1. — *Ileum atresia.*

A. — UNDERDEVELOPMENT

— *Agenesis* or complete absence of an intestinal segment, clearly incompatible with survival when it is very extensive.

— *Atresia* (fig. 1): an intestinal segment is, and remains, very narrow and constricted; passage of food is obstructed.

— *Aplasia,* where the contracted segment nevertheless has a mucosa and a lumen.

— *Mucosal narrowing,* often associated with other anomalies.

B. — OVERDEVELOPMENT

— *Duplications,* ranging from the simple diverticulum to almost complete doubling of the digestive tube, including many varieties of cystic malformations. Their common component is their localization on the mesenteric (that is, dorsal) border of the intestine.

C. — ABNORMAL PERSISTENCE OF EMBRYONIC STRUCTURES

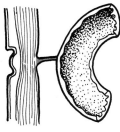

Ligament.

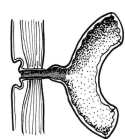

Umbilical fistula.

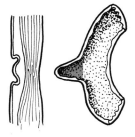

Typical diverticulum.

Fig. 2.

Most frequent types of Meckel's diverticulum.

— *Meckel's diverticulum* (fig. 2). — The most well known of this type of malformation. It involves a remnant of the vitelline duct and may occur in multiple anatomic forms: complete duct, full cord, intermediate cysts, blind fistula, and, most often, simple intestinal diverticulum. It must be emphasized that the mucosa lining these formations may be of the gastric, rather than intestinal, type, which explains part of the complications (ulcers, hemorrhages). The diverticulum, or its equivalent, is always located on the antimesenteric (that is, ventral) side of the intestine.

MALFORMATIONS

— **Dorsal intestinal fistulas.** These may be due to an abnormal adherence of the entoderm to the ectoderm. Persistance of this abnormal condition leads, during gastrulation, to doubling of the notochord and more or less apparent anomalies of neural tube closure. Here, again, all degrees are possible: total fistula, cysts, cords, etc.

II. — ANOMALIES OF POSITION

In addition to complete absence of rotation, and all varieties of incomplete rotation involving an isolated segment, there are also rotations in opposite direction to normal; mirror-image rotation, or clockwise rotation (retroduodenal colon).

III. — ANOMALIES OF MESENTERIC ATTACHMENT

Between total absence of attachment (persistence of common mesentery), and excessive attachment, all intermediate forms can be seen. All may remain completely latent, or reveal themselves abruptly by a change in digestive transport.

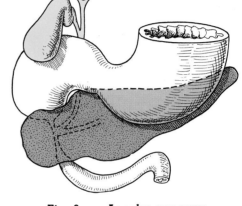

Fig. 3. — *Annular pancreas.*

IV. — EXTRINSIC COMPRESSION

Annular pancreas is an example of this type of anomaly (fig. 3). It is caused by failure of the ventral pancreatic bud to migrate, or by the presence of a supernumerary bud. The ring of pancreatic tissue thus formed may constrict the duodenum and cause obstructions in the newborn (see p. 35).

V. — HISTOLOGICAL ANOMALIES

Aganglionic dystony. — Also called Hirschsprung's disease, this condition may affect the colon, the small intestine or the duodenum, but especially the rectum. The gravity of the disease is directly proportional to the length of the segment affected, and results from functional alteration as well as cytologic abnormality of the nerve plexes of the intestinal wall.

— **Mucoviscidosis:** adherence of meconium to the intestinal wall, secondary to a deficiency of trypsin secretion by the pancreas, which is invaded by interstitial fibrosis of unknown origin.

Omphalocele, often included among digestive anomalies, is actually a malformation of the anterior body wall. It is, however, often associated with anomalies of union of the digestive tube.

HINDGUT

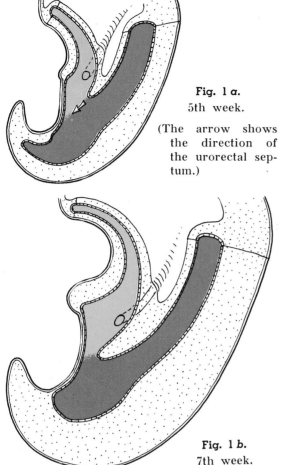

Fig. 1 a.
5th week.

(The arrow shows the direction of the urorectal septum.)

Fig. 1 b.
7th week.

SUBDIVISION OF CLOACA

The hindgut follows the midgut and gives rise to the left third of the transverse colon, the descending colon, the sigmoid, and the rectum. Its distal portion participates in formation of the *cloaca*.

— At its cephalic end, the cloaca is continuous with the allantois, and at its caudal end with the tail gut.

— Ventrally, the entodermal lining of the cloaca is in direct contact with the surface ectoderm, without interposition of mesenchyme: this forms the *cloacal membrane*.

— Between the precloacal hindgut and the allantois, a mesenchymal projection is formed, covered with entoderm. This is the *urorectal septum,* which divides the arch of the cloaca.

— Later, the cloaca receives the Wolffian ducts which open cranially and ventrally to the projection of the urorectal septum (fig. 1 *a*).

From the end of the 5th week to the 7th week, the urorectal septum elongates in the direction of the cloacal membrane (fig. 1 *a* and *b*). It reaches the membrane during the 8th week (fig. 1 *c*).

— The cloaca is thus divided into the rectum posteriorly, and the urogenital sinus anteriorly. The latter receives on its posterior side the two Wolffian ducts.

— The cloacal membrane is subdivided into the *urogenital membrane* anteriorly, and the *anal membrane* posteriorly. Between these two transitory membranes, the mesenchyme of the urorectal septum covered with surface ectoderm forms the *perineum*.

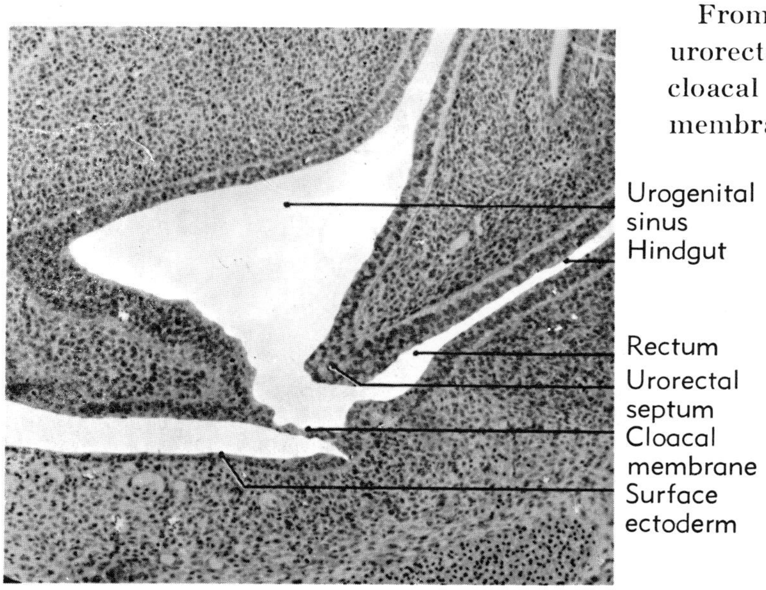

Urogenital sinus
Hindgut

Rectum
Urorectal septum
Cloacal membrane
Surface ectoderm

Fig. 2. — *Cloaca in process of septation.*
Sagittal median section.
Rabbit embryo, 8 days (× 110).

RECTUM AND ANAL MEMBRANE

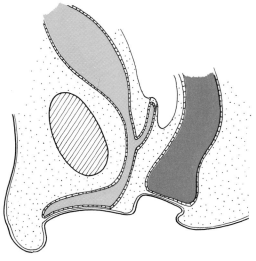

Fig. 1 c. — 8th week.

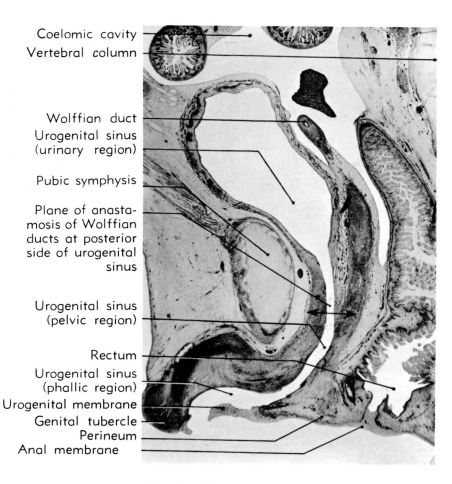

Coelomic cavity
Vertebral column

Wolffian duct
Urogenital sinus
(urinary region)

Pubic symphysis

Plane of anasta-
mosis of Wolffian
ducts at posterior
side of urogenital
sinus

Urogenital sinus
(pelvic region)

Rectum
Urogenital sinus
(phallic region)
Urogenital membrane
Genital tubercle
Perineum
Anal membrane

Fig. 4. — *Rectum and urogenital sinus.* Human fetus at 9th week. Sagittal section of pelvic region (× 15).

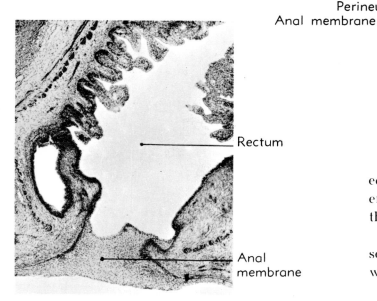

Rectum

Anal
membrane

Fig. 3. — *Anal membrane.*
Sagittal section,
9th week fetus (× 35).

In the ninth week, the anal membrane is in an ectodermal depression connected with the mesenchymal proliferation of the adjacent area: this is the proctodeum or future anal canal.

Soon thereafter, the anal membrane is resorbed, allowing communication of the rectum with the anal canal.

This embryonic configuration explains the presence of the stratified squamous epithelium in the anal canal, as opposed to the glandular epithelium in the rectum.

A. — **Clinically,** there are three major types of anorectal malformations:

— *Imperforate anus* (absent anus). This is classical *anal imperforation,* and includes many varieties which all require immediate surgical treatment.

— *Insufficient anus*—leads to problems of meconial evacuation and should be treated without delay.

— *Ectopic anus*—slightly less serious, for it permits some intestinal transport, but is always functionally insufficient.

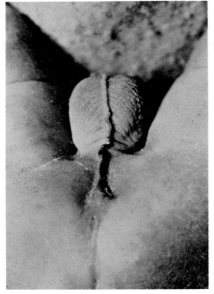

Fig. 1. — *Imperforate (covered) anus with scrotal fistula* (courtesy of Dr. B. DUHAMEL).

B. — **Embryologically,** it seems preferable to differentiate:

1. **Superficial malformations,** due to anomalies in formation and fixation of superficial perineal levels. In this class are insufficient anus, covered anus (membranous imperforation), and covered anus with fistula (fig. 1 and 2).

2. **Deep malformations,** where the anomaly affects septation of the cloaca by aberrant migration of the urorectal septum. It may involve:

— *pure rectal atresia,* complete failure of formation of the inferior portion of the rectum and the anal canal (fig. 3);

— *rectal atresia with fistula* (always insufficient). Length and degree of anastomosis differentiates the various types of this anomaly (fig. 4 and 5).

3. **Mixed malformations,** including all forms of ectopic anus. These abnormal anastomoses of the anus to the perineum reflect both perineal and cloacal abnormalities. They seriously affect function, although less severely than the two preceding groups.

MALFORMATIONS

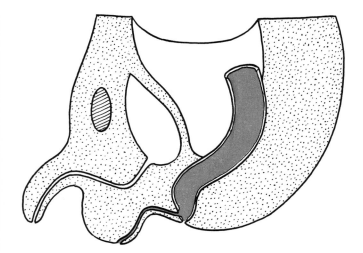

Fig. 2. — *Impertorate anus with scrotal fistula.*

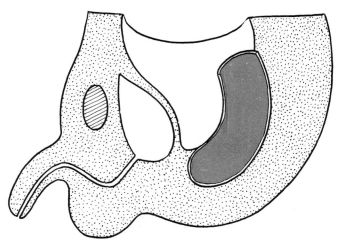

Fig. 3. — *Rectal atresia.*

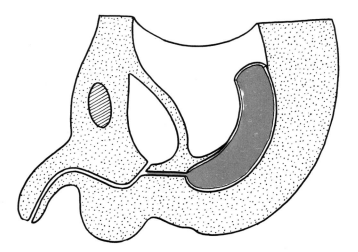

Fig. 4. — *Rectal atresia with urinary fistula.*

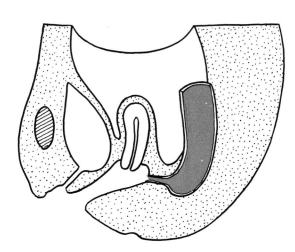

Fig. 5. — *Rectal atresia with vaginal fistula.*

RESPIRATORY

TRACHEOBRONCHIAL

Development of the respiratory system begins in the embryo at about the 3 mm stage, toward the end of the 3rd week. By the 6th month, the lung has developed sufficiently to insure viability.

Like the digestive tube from which it derives, the respiratory system has a double origin:

— *entodermic:* tracheobronchial epithelium, alveolar endothelium, accessory glands;

— *mesodermic:* chorion, cartilaginous structures, smooth muscle, and vascular system.

The beginning of respiratory system development is marked by longitudinal evagination on the anterior side of the foregut, below the pharyngeal gut. This is the *tracheal groove* (fig. 1 and 2).

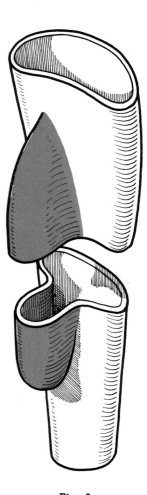

Fig. 2.
Tracheal groove.

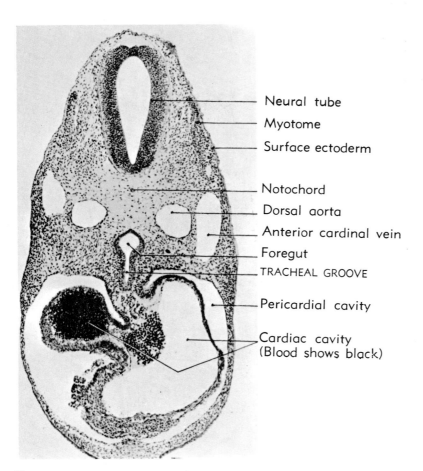

- Neural tube
- Myotome
- Surface ectoderm

- Notochord
- Dorsal aorta
- Anterior cardinal vein
- Foregut
- TRACHEAL GROOVE

- Pericardial cavity

- Cardiac cavity (Blood shows black)

Fig. 1. — *Tracheal groove.* Cross section of thoracic region. Rabbit embryo, 8th day (× 65).

This groove is progressively separated from the digestive tube by a process of lateral pinching off which proceeds in the caudocephalic direction (fig. 4).

Thus, the trachea ventrally, and the esophagus dorsally, are differentiated.

SYSTEM

DEVELOPMENT

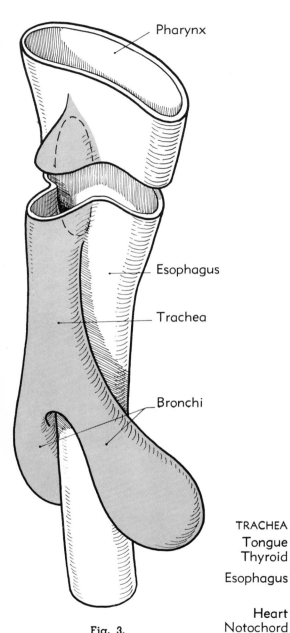

Pharynx

Esophagus

Trachea

Bronchi

Fig. 3.
Primitive tracheobronchial tree.

The trachea elongates caudally and bifurcates into two lateral stumps, *the lung buds,* or *primary tracheal buds.*

The trachea remains open in the foregut at the laryngeal orifice (or glottis).

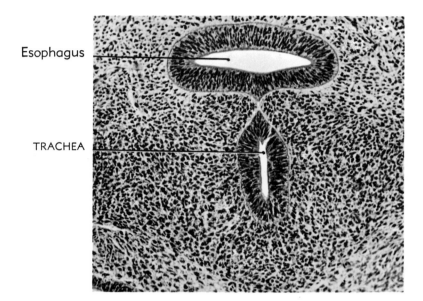

Esophagus

TRACHEA

Fig. 4. — *Separation of the trachea is almost finished.* Cross section of thoracic region. Human embryo, 4.2 mm (× 180).

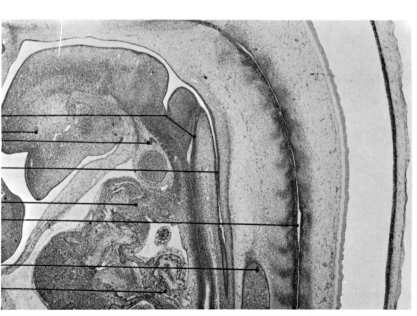

TRACHEA
Tongue
Thyroid

Esophagus

Heart
Notochord

Aorta
Venous sinus

Fig. 5. — *Definitive trachea and esophagus.*
Sagittal median section of cervicothoracic region.
Rabbit embryo, 14 days (× 25).

The *lung buds,* arising at the caudal end of the trachea, penetrate the neighboring mesenchyme. They branch further by successive division into smaller and smaller bronchi until the 6th month. This bronchial tree, covered with mesenchyme, projects into the upper part of the coelomic cavity, the future pleural cavity. These are the pulmonary primordia, initially supplied by numerous vessels mainly aortic in origin.

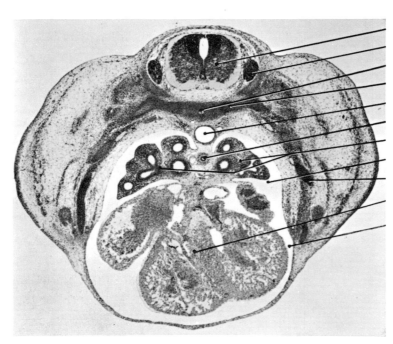

Spinal cord
Spinal ganglion
Notochord
Sclerotome
Aorta
Esophagus
Pulmonary primordia
Pleural cavity
Ribs
Heart
Pericardial cavity

Fig. 1. — *Pulmonary primordia.*
Cross section. Thorax. Rat embryo, 15 days (× 25).

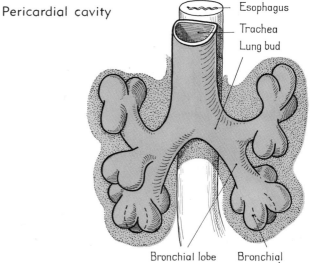

Esophagus
Trachea
Lung bud

Bronchial lobe   Bronchial segment

Fig. 3. — *Lung buds.*

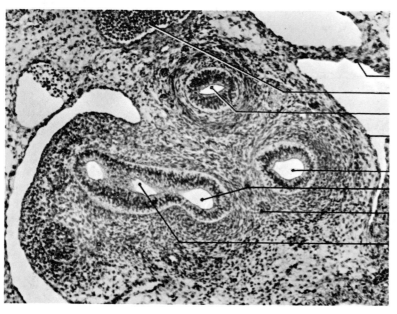

Parietal pleura
Aorta

Esophagus

Visceral pleura

LEFT LUNG BUD

RIGHT LUNG BUD

Mesenchyme

Origin of the right upper bronchial lobe

Fig. 2. — *Lung primordia* of a 34-day human embryo. Cross section (× 110). Note the similarity at this stage of the esophageal and bronchial epithelia.

PULMONARY PRIMORDIA

About the 5th month, branches of the pulmonary artery and alveoli develop simultaneously at the end of each bronchiole. By the 6th month, the respiratory system is complete and its control centers are mature. From now on, the fetus is viable.

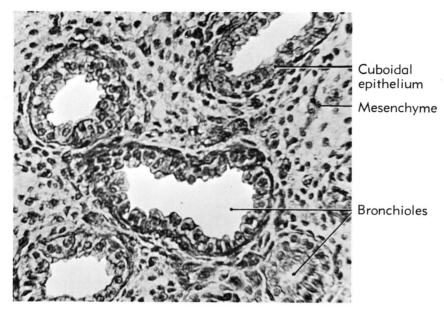

Cuboidal epithelium

Mesenchyme

Bronchioles

Fig. 4. — *Bronchiolar stage.*
Pulmonary parenchyma
of 3-month human fetus (× 300).

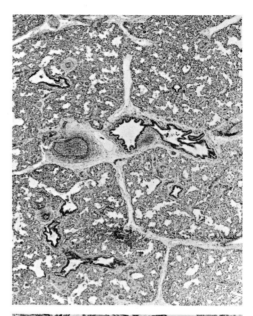

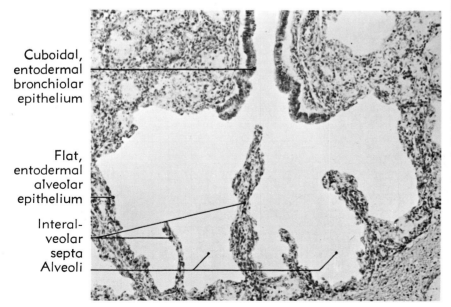

Cuboidal, entodermal bronchiolar epithelium

Flat, entodermal alveolar epithelium

Interal-veolar septa
Alveoli

Fig. 5. — *Pulmonary alveoli.* Human fetus of 7 months
(× 100). Epithelium of the bronchi and of the alveoli,
although of the same origin, are clearly different.

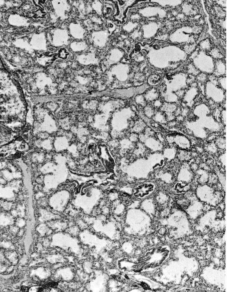

Fig. 6. — *Upper*: Lung from 9-month human fetus which has not respired. Alveoli collapsed.

Lower: Lung of newborn after respiration; the alveoli are expanded.

Both photographs are at same enlargement (× 10).

The major respiratory system malformations can be classified into four groups.

I. — BRONCHIAL ANOMALIES DUE TO FAILURE OF LUNG BUD TO DEVELOP

Agenesis is indicated by total absence of the bronchial tree, alveolar tissue and vascular system. Bilateral agenesis, with the trachea terminating in a blind end, is unusual. In unilateral agenesis, there is no lung bud on the affected side. Partial agenesis also occurs; this may be lobar, segmental, or bronchiolar.

Aplasia is unilateral as a rule, and differs from similar agenesis by the presence of a stump of the lung bud.

Hypoplasia is characterized by insufficient development. It may be total, involving an entire lung, or partial, concerning only a restricted region.

II. — BRONCHIAL ANOMALIES DUE TO MALPOSITION

Three types can be distinguished:
— *bronchial variations,* where the abnormality involves only division of the bronchopulmonary tree. These are very frequent;
— *abnormalities of bronchial division:* supernumerary bronchi and lungs;
— *abnormalities of symmetry:* situs inversus and mirror-image lungs.

III. — ANOMALIES DUE TO "BRONCHIAL DETACHMENT" OR SEQUESTRATION

These abnormalities of bronchopulmonary tissue may:
— retain normal appearance, although the alveoli are not expanded; or
— more often, show clear predominance of bronchial structures with cysts.
The sequestrations are most often intralobar, but sometimes extralobar, and have 2 essential characteristics.

a) Their vascularization is systemic, coming directly from the aorta or one of its collaterals. There is no blood supplied by the pulmonary artery.

b) Their bronchi are not part of the tracheobronchial tree.

Whatever may be their origin, such cystic structures result in those parts of a lung being badly, or not at all, ventilated. Also because of their abnormal vascularization, they cannot participate in oxygenation of blood.

OF RESPIRATORY SYSTEM

IV. — FAILURE OF CLEAVAGE OF TRACHEAL GROOVE: ESOPHAGEAL ATRESIA AND ESOPHAGEOTRACHEAL FISTULAS

Esophageotracheal fistulas are caused by incomplete separation between the esophagus and the trachea at the time of cleavage of the esophageotracheal groove, during the 4th week of development. Fistulas almost always accompany esophageal atresia.

Without a fistula, the esophageotracheal septum encroaches excessively on the esophageal lumen and brings about isolated esophageal atresia.

Frequency of these malformations is about 1 in 2,500 births.

According to Ladd, there are *5 anatomic types.*

— Types 3 and 4, shown in the box in the diagram below, are by far the most frequent, 95% of all cases: esophageotracheal or esophageobronchial fistula on the lower part of the esophagus, below the atresia.

— Type 5 is rather rare: double fistula, surrounding the atresia.

— Types 1 and 2, simple esophageal atresia, without fistula, and esophageal atresia with fistula above, are extremely rare.

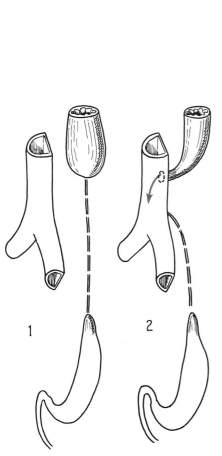

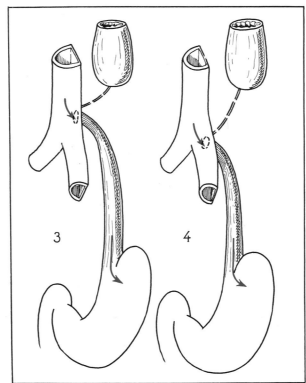

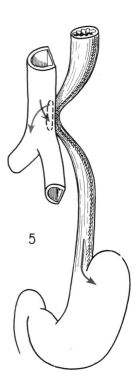

Ladd's Classification.

In types 3, 4, and 5, the blue arrow shows passage of air in the digestive tract. A standard X-ray picture showing air in the abdomen, thus allows elimination of types 1 and 2.

INTERMEDIATE PLATE

The urinary system is derived from the intermediate mesoderm between the paraxial (somite-forming) mesoderm and the lateral plate.

Its development takes place in the craniocaudal direction in successive chronological steps.

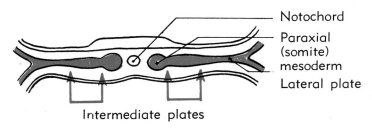

Fig. 1. — *Diagram of embryo at 3 germinal layer stage.*

The definitive kidney, or **metanephros,** is preceded by two transitory structures.

— **The pronephros** may be thought of as a rough draft and is rapidly replaced.

— **The mesonephros** attains complete development, but later mostly regresses. Its remnants are incorporated into the urogenital system.

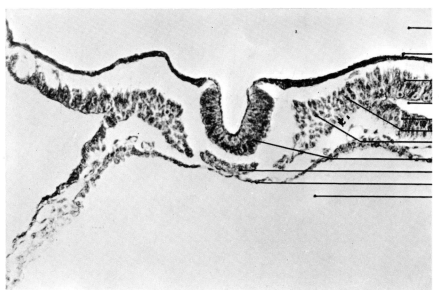

Fig. 2. — *Intraembryonic mesoderm.*
Rabbit embryo, 8 1/2 days. Cross section (× 145).

SYSTEM

NEPHROGENIC CORD

The nephrogenic cord is first continuous with the somite (paraxial) mesoderm internally, and the lateral plate externally. Later, it separates, while remaining very close to the intraembryonic coelom. Like the somite mesoderm, it undergoes grossly metameric segmentation, into nephrotomes.

This metamerization is clear at the cranial end, but only rudimentary in the middle portion of the embryo, and practically nonexistent at the caudal end, where the nephrogenic mesoderm remains undivided.

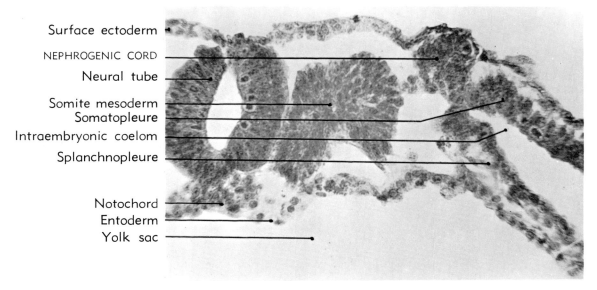

Surface ectoderm
NEPHROGENIC CORD
Neural tube
Somite mesoderm
Somatopleure
Intraembryonic coelom
Splanchnopleure

Notochord
Entoderm
Yolk sac

Fig. 3. — *Nephrogenic cord.*
Rabbit embryo, 9 days. Cross section ($\times$ 280).

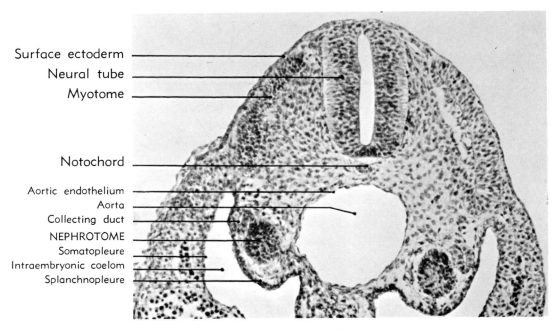

Surface ectoderm
Neural tube
Myotome

Notochord

Aortic endothelium
Aorta
Collecting duct
NEPHROTOME
Somatopleure
Intraembryonic coelom
Splanchnopleure

Fig. 4. — *Nephrotome.*
Rabbit embryo, 10 days. Cross section ($\times$ 145).

DEVELOPMENT OF NEPHROGENIC CORD

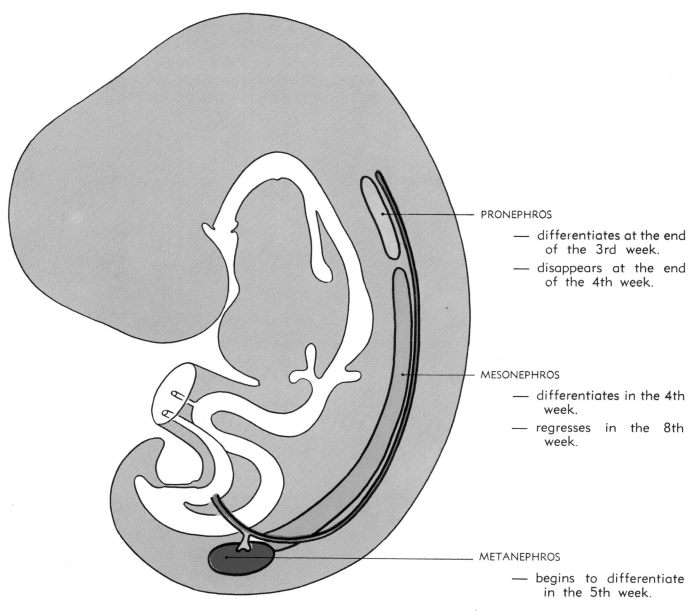

PRONEPHROS

— differentiates at the end of the 3rd week.

— disappears at the end of the 4th week.

MESONEPHROS

— differentiates in the 4th week.

— regresses in the 8th week.

METANEPHROS

— begins to differentiate in the 5th week.

Fig. 1. — *The three kidneys.*

The 3 primordia are shown together, although in reality they succeed each other.
The secretory and excretory parts, *although of the same origin,* are shown in different colors.

These three primordia succeed each other, not only in time but in space, arising from the long ribbon of nephrogenic cord which differentiates progressively from the cervical to the caudal region.

PRONEPHROS

21 days

28 days

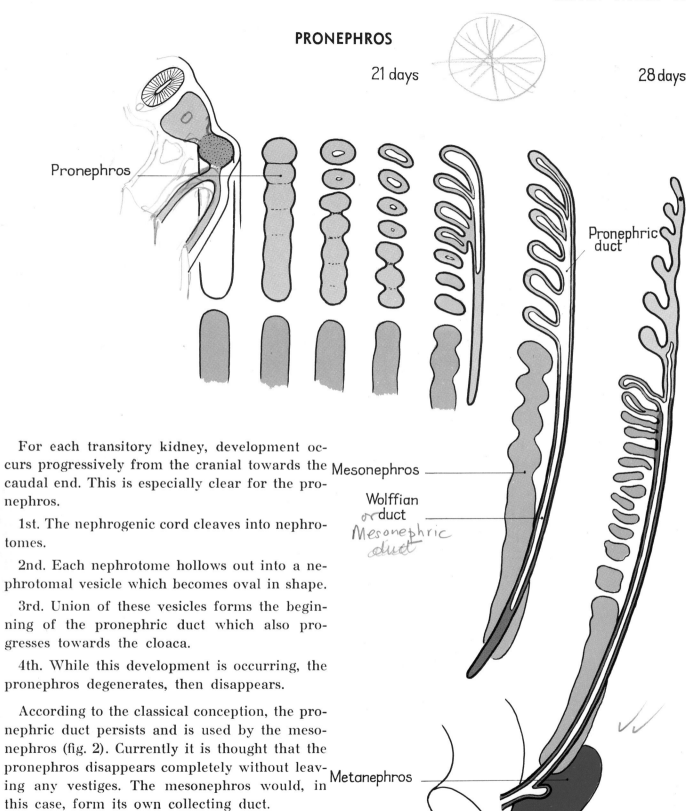

Pronephros

Pronephric duct

Mesonephros

Wolffian or duct

Mesonephric duct

Metanephros

For each transitory kidney, development occurs progressively from the cranial towards the caudal end. This is especially clear for the pronephros.

1st. The nephrogenic cord cleaves into nephrotomes.

2nd. Each nephrotome hollows out into a nephrotomal vesicle which becomes oval in shape.

3rd. Union of these vesicles forms the beginning of the pronephric duct which also progresses towards the cloaca.

4th. While this development is occurring, the pronephros degenerates, then disappears.

According to the classical conception, the pronephric duct persists and is used by the mesonephros (fig. 2). Currently it is thought that the pronephros disappears completely without leaving any vestiges. The mesonephros would, in this case, form its own collecting duct.

Fig. 2. — *Development of the pronephros* (according to the classical conception).

MESONEPHROS

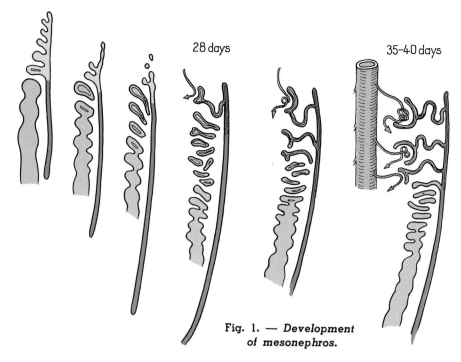

28 days   35-40 days

Fig. 1. — *Development of mesonephros.*

As in development of the pronephros, the mesonephric nephrotomes pass through the following stages, beginning the 4th week:
— solid nephrotome;
— nephrotomal vesicle;
— lengthening of vesicle into tubule;
— enlargement of its internal end into a glomerular chamber opposite an arterial loop coming from the aorta;
— arrangement of the glomerular chamber around an arterial capillary cluster;
— opening of the tubule into the mesonephric or Wolffian duct (which may or may not be preexistent as the pronephric duct).

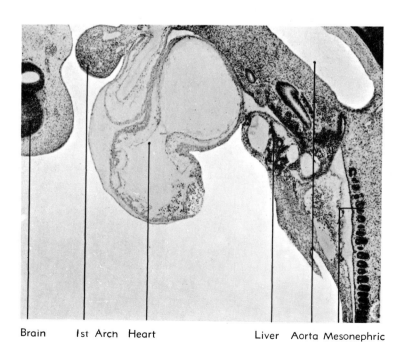

Brain   1st Arch Heart   Liver Aorta Mesonephric
                                              vesicles

Fig. 2. — *Mesonephric vesicles.*
Rabbit embryo, 11 days. Sagittal section (× 35).

*Figures 2 and 3 represent equivalent stages
and are at the same enlargement.*

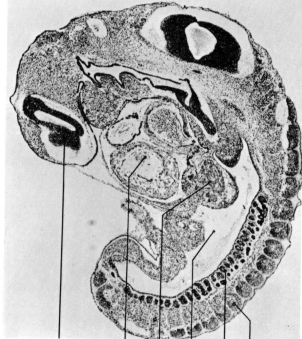

Brain   Heart Liver Body Meso Somites
                       cavity nephros

Fig. 3. — *Mesonephric vesicles.* Note the dorsolumbar location. Human embryo. Section is very oblique in relation to embryonic axis.

OR WOLFFIAN BODY

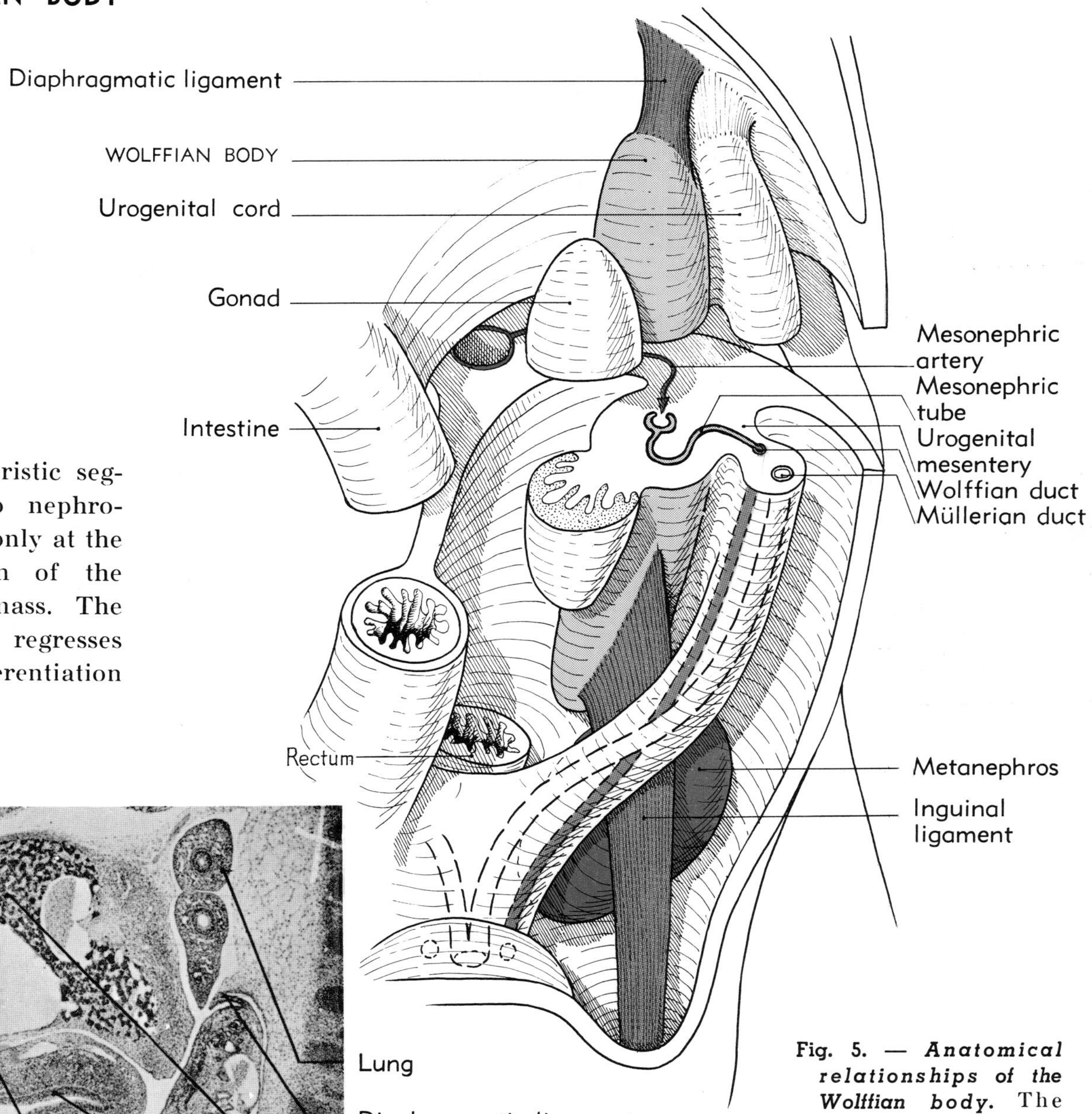

Diaphragmatic ligament

WOLFFIAN BODY

Urogenital cord

Gonad

Intestine

The characteristic segmentation into nephrotomes is clear only at the cranial portion of the mesonephric mass. The caudal portion regresses before its differentiation is complete.

Rectum

Mesonephric artery
Mesonephric tube
Urogenital mesentery
Wolffian duct
Müllerian duct

Metanephros

Inguinal ligament

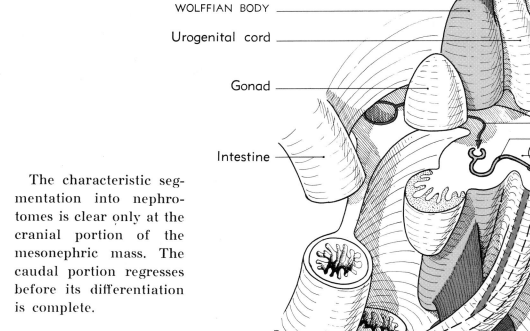

Fig. 5. — *Anatomical relationships of the Wolffian body.* The gonadal primordium develops at its anterior internal side.

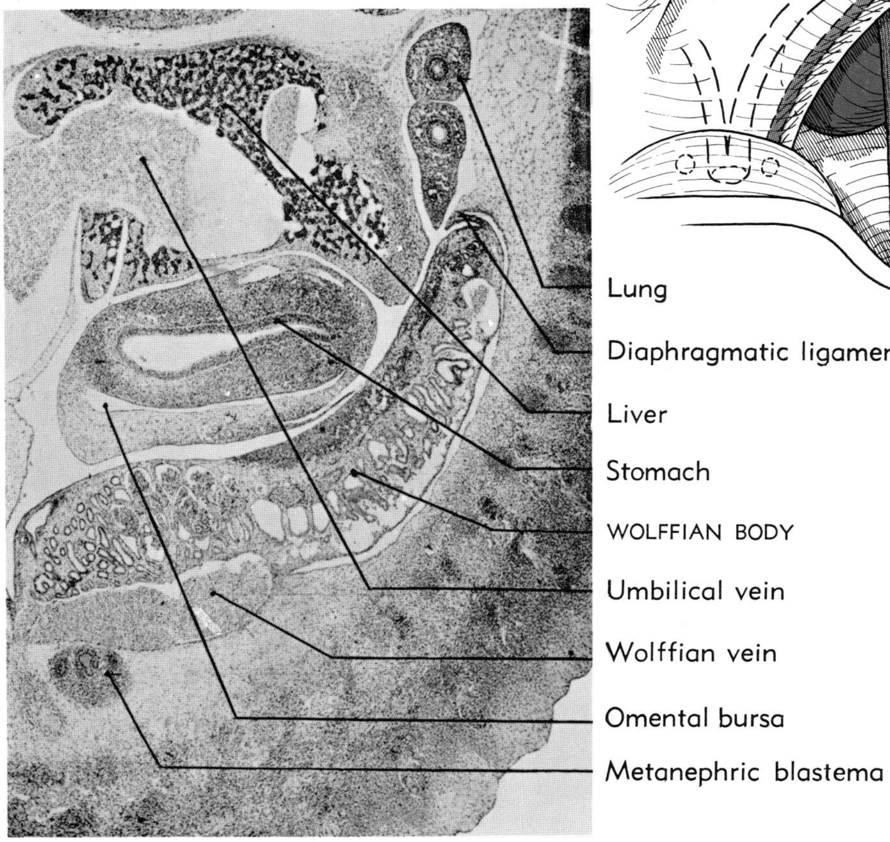

Lung

Diaphragmatic ligament

Liver

Stomach

WOLFFIAN BODY

Umbilical vein

Wolffian vein

Omental bursa

Metanephric blastema

Fig. 4.
Wolffian body. Rabbit embryo, 14 days. Paramedial sagittal section of abdomen ($\times$ 30).

In cross section, the Wolffian body appears to be a mass projecting into the peritoneal cavity.

On its anteroexternal edge, attached by the *urogenital mesentery*, is the *urogenital cord* containing the Wolffian and Müllerian ducts.

On its anterointernal side is the *gonadal primordium*, attached by the *gonadal mesentery*.

Its posterior face is attached to the dorsal body wall by the *Wolffian body mesentery*, which is wide and close to the root of the mesentery, beside the aorta. The coelomic epithelium inside this mesentery is the origin of the adrenal cortex (fig. 1 and 3).

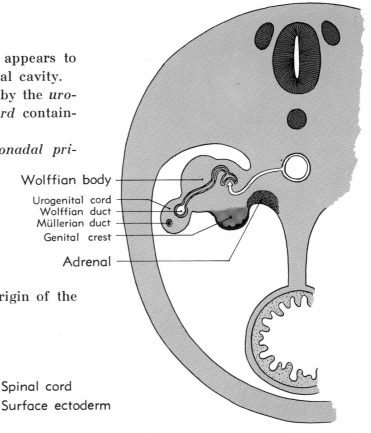

Wolffian body
Urogenital cord
Wolffian duct
Müllerian duct
Genital crest
Adrenal

Fig. 1. — *Relationship of Wolffian body with gonadal and adrenal primordia.*
Diagram of a cross section.

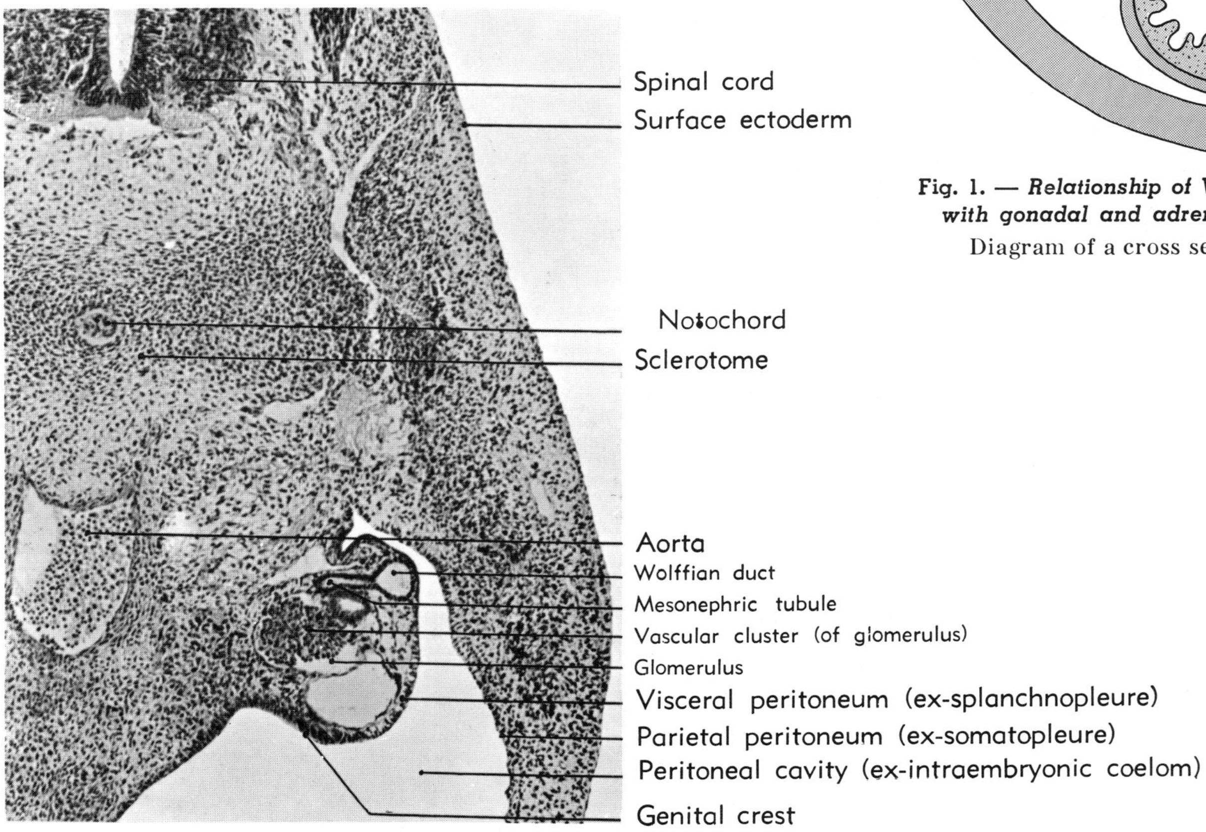

Spinal cord
Surface ectoderm

Notochord
Sclerotome

Aorta
Wolffian duct
Mesonephric tubule
Vascular cluster (of glomerulus)
Glomerulus
Visceral peritoneum (ex-splanchnopleure)
Parietal peritoneum (ex-somatopleure)
Peritoneal cavity (ex-intraembryonic coelom)
Genital crest

Fig. 2. — *Wolffian body.*
Human embryo, 4.2 mm.
Cross section of abdomen (× 60).

OF MESONEPHROS

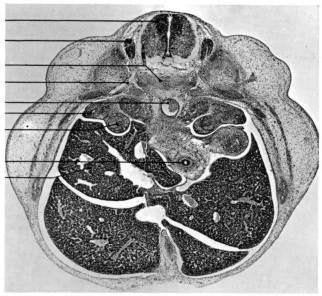

Spinal cord
Spinal ganglion
Notochord surrounded by sclerotome
Mixed nerve
Aorta
Wolffian body
Gonad
Esophagus
Liver

Fig. 3. — *Lumbar region.*
Cross section.   Rat embryo, 15 days (× 25).

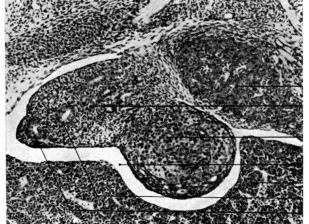

Adrenal
Wolffian body
and mesonephric tubules
Gonad

Peritoneal cavity
Liver
Wolffian duct
Müllerian duct

Fig. 4. — *Wolffian body.*
Gonad and adrenal (× 100).

Parietal peritoneum
Visceral peritoneum

Wolffian duct, receiving
mesonephric tubules
Müllerian duct

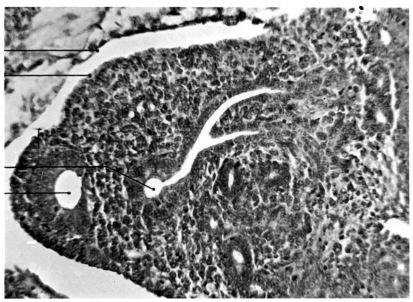

These 3 sections of the same embryo, at increasing enlargement, illustrate the relationships and constituents of the Wolffian body.

Fig. 5. — *Wolffian body* (× 260).

REGRESSION OF WOLFFIAN BODY

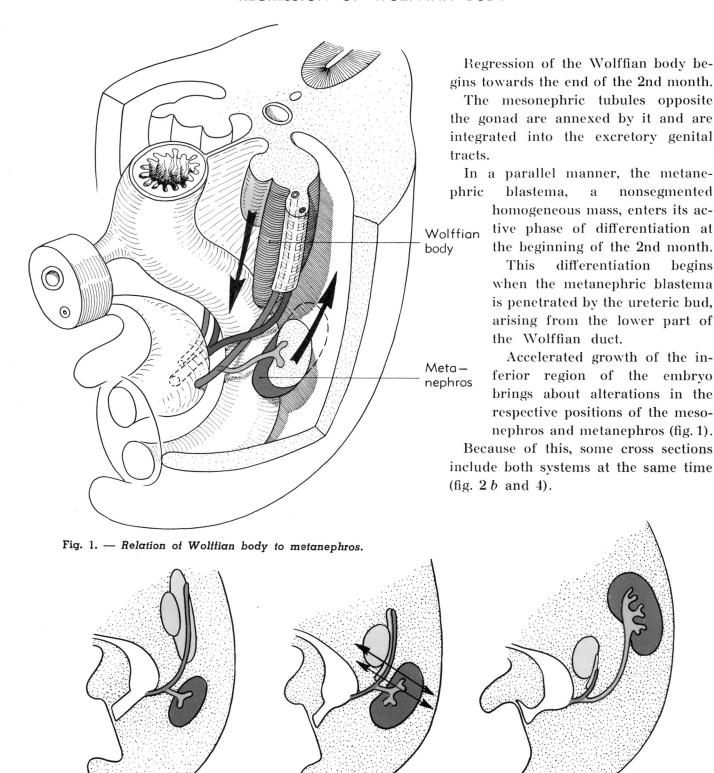

Regression of the Wolffian body begins towards the end of the 2nd month.

The mesonephric tubules opposite the gonad are annexed by it and are integrated into the excretory genital tracts.

In a parallel manner, the metanephric blastema, a nonsegmented homogeneous mass, enters its active phase of differentiation at the beginning of the 2nd month.

This differentiation begins when the metanephric blastema is penetrated by the ureteric bud, arising from the lower part of the Wolffian duct.

Accelerated growth of the inferior region of the embryo brings about alterations in the respective positions of the mesonephros and metanephros (fig. 1).

Because of this, some cross sections include both systems at the same time (fig. 2 b and 4).

Wolffian body

Meta—
nephros

Fig. 1. — *Relation of Wolffian body to metanephros.*

5th week

8th week

After the 2nd month

a

b

c

Fig. 2. — *Stages of development of mesonephros and metanephros.*

DIFFERENTIATION OF METANEPHROS

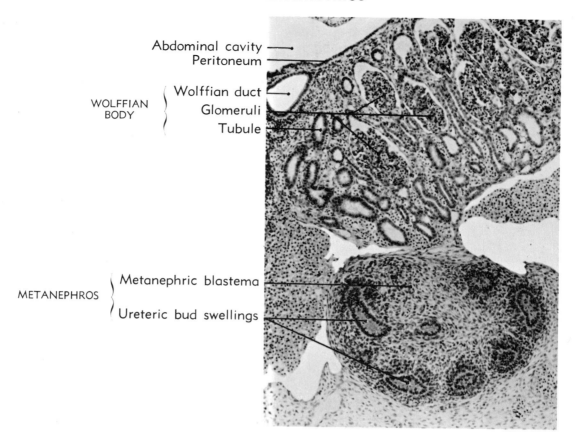

Abdominal cavity
Peritoneum

WOLFFIAN
BODY
}
Wolffian duct
Glomeruli
Tubule

METANEPHROS
}
Metanephric blastema
Ureteric bud swellings

Fig. 3. — *Wolffian body and initial stage of metanephros.* Rabbit embryo, 14 days (× 100). Paramedian sagittal section.

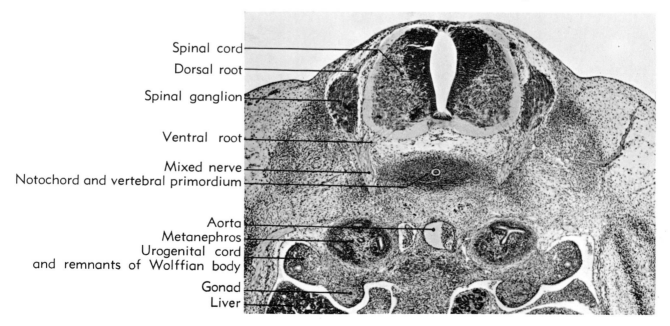

Spinal cord
Dorsal root

Spinal ganglion

Ventral root

Mixed nerve
Notochord and vertebral primordium

Aorta
Metanephros
Urogenital cord
and remnants of Wolffian body
Gonad
Liver

Fig. 4. — *More developed metanephros, with ureteric bud.* Cross section. Rat embryo, 15 days (× 50). At level shown by upper arrow in diagram 2 *b*.

URETERIC BUD

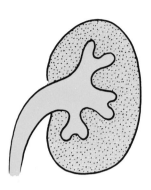

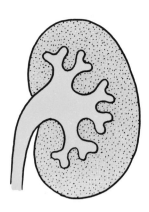

Fig. 1. — *Penetration of blastema by ureteric bud.*

The ureteric bud arises at the beginning of the 2nd month, from the lower end of the Wolffian duct. It rapidly reaches and penetrates the metanephric blastema. It then enlarges, forming the beginning of the *renal pelvis* (5 weeks) with two diverticula, one cranial and one caudal.

The renal pelvis then gives rise to *tubules* which penetrate further into the metanephric mass (fig. 1).

These in turn further subdivide, and in the process compress the blastema eccentrically (fig. 2).

The ducts continue to subdivide until 15 generations of ducts have been formed.

A complete system of branching ducts, forming a renal lobe, result from each tubule of the first generation.

Then these first generation tubules enlarge and incorporate the later tubules up to the 6th generation (fig. 3).

In this way are formed the *calyces,* into which the papillary ducts empty (fig. 4).

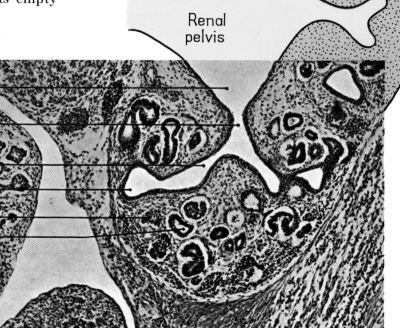

Renal pelvis

1st generation tubule

2nd generation tubule

3rd generation tubule

Metanephric spheroids
Metanephric vesicles

Fig. 2. — *Branching of ureteric bud in blastema.*

Section of metanephros. Human fetus, 2 1/4 months (× 110).

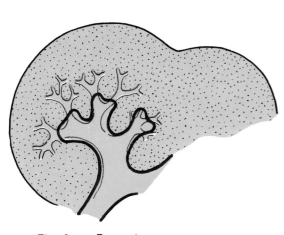

Fig. 3. — *Formation of the calyces.*

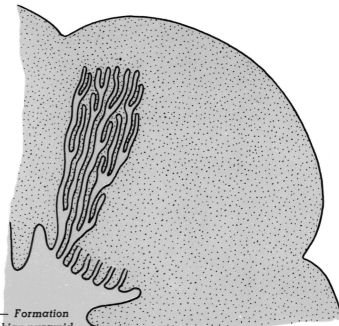

Fig. 4. — *Formation of Malpighian pyramid.*

The ureteric duct thus gives rise to the entire **collecting system** of the kidney: ureter, renal pelvis, calyces, papillary ducts, and collecting tubules.

The metanephric blastema gives rise to the entire **excretory system.**

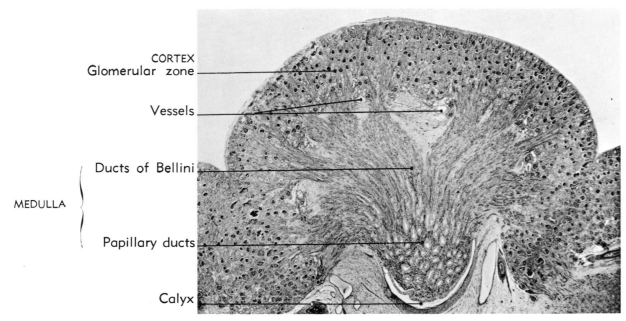

Fig. 5. — *Definitive appearance of Malpighian pyramid.*
Kidney of human fetus, 3 1/2 months (× 16).

The tubular branching derived from the ureteric bud penetrates the metanephric blastema, compressing it eccentrically, and fragmenting it into tissue caps.

At each end of the cap, a metanephric spheroid arises which undergoes the same transformations as those already seen for the nephrotomes of the pronephros and mesonephros.

Here, however, differentiation is much more elaborate, leading to formation of *functional units.*

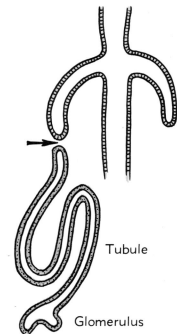

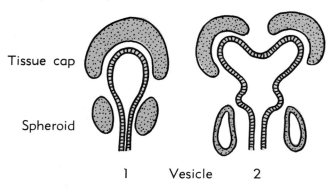

Tissue cap

Spheroid

1   Vesicle   2

3

Tubule

Glomerulus

4

Fig. 1. — *Development of metanephric blastema.* 1. spheroid stage; 2. vesicle stage; 3. the vesicle elongates in an S shape; and 4. finally opens into the collecting tubule.

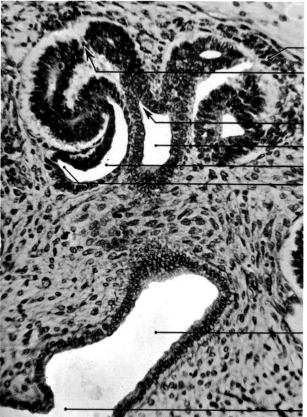

Metanephric cap

Region of junction of excretory and collecting portions

Future collecting duct

End of a 6th order tubule

Vesicle

Region of future glomerulus

5th order tubule

Renal pelvis

The number of functional units grows by concentric layers throughout prenatal life.

Fig. 2. — *Excretory and collecting systems of definitive kidney.*

Renal parenchyma of a human fetus, 2 1/4 months ($\times$ 240).

BLASTEMA

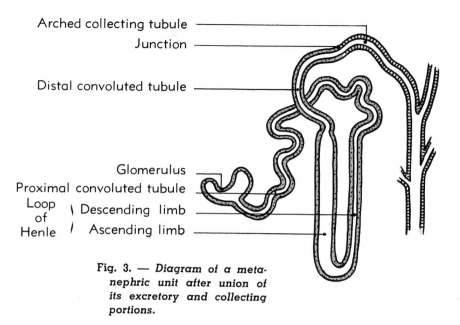

Arched collecting tubule

Junction

Distal convoluted tubule

Glomerulus
Proximal convoluted tubule
Loop of Henle { Descending limb / Ascending limb

Fig. 3. — *Diagram of a metanephric unit after union of its excretory and collecting portions.*

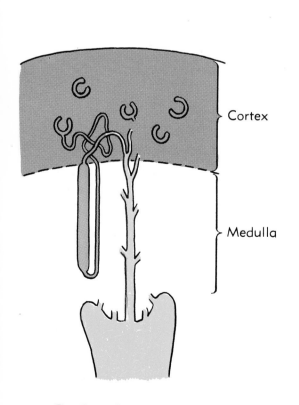

Cortex

Medulla

Fig. 5. — *Arrangement of definitive functional unit from the 3rd month on.*

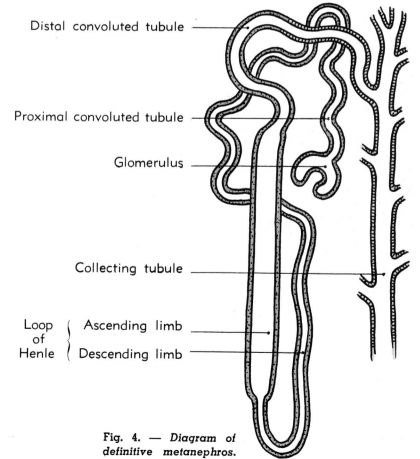

Distal convoluted tubule

Proximal convoluted tubule

Glomerulus

Collecting tubule

Loop of Henle { Ascending limb / Descending limb

Fig. 4. — *Diagram of definitive metanephros.*

CORTEX {
Renal capsule
Glomerulus
Proximal convoluted tubules

MEDULLA {
Loop of Henle {
Descending limb
Ascending limb

Tuge of Bellini
Loop of Henle

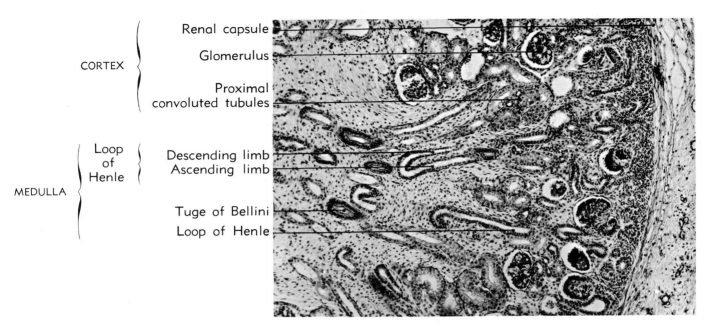

Fig. 1. — *Definitive renal parenchyma.*
Kidney of human fetus, 3 months (× 90).

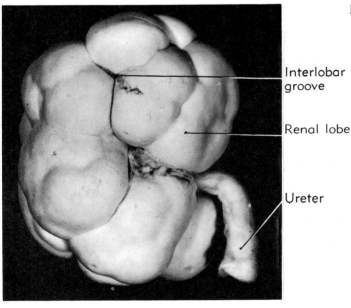

Interlobar groove

Renal lobe

Ureter

Fig. 2. — *Fetal kidney with characteristic lobes.*
Human fetus, 4 months.

The fetal kidney normally has a polylobar appearance due to the particular manner of development of the ureteric bud in the metanephric blastema.

This lobular form is diminished at the time of birth through progressive filling in of the interlobular grooves. The adult kidney is smooth and regular. Sometimes, however, the prenatal appearance persists, and is then called a *polylobed kidney*.

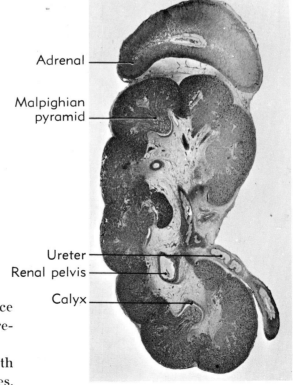

Adrenal

Malpighian pyramid

Ureter
Renal pelvis

Calyx

Fig. 3. — *Longitudinal section. Kidney and adrenal.* Kidney of human fetus, 3 1/2 months (× 3.5).

KIDNEY

The two photographs below show that by the 3rd month, the nephrons already formed are anatomically and histologically identical to those of the adult kidney. At this stage, the kidney begins to manufacture urine. However, it has still not acquired its total number of functional units (of the order of one million). Some of these units are not formed until about term, or perhaps even in some cases, after birth.

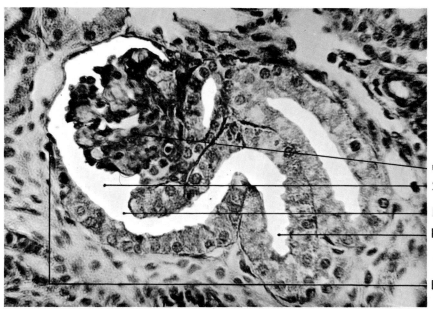

Glomerulus

Subcapsular space

Neck

Proximal convoluted tubule

Bowman's capsule

Fig. 4. — *Urinary aspect of glomerulus.*
Kidney of human fetus, 3 months (× 590).

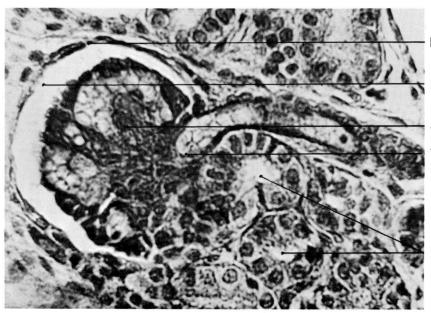

Bowman's capsule

Subcapsular space

Glomerular vascular tuft

Vascular pole
(afferent and efferent capillaries)

Proximal convoluted tubules

Fig. 5. — *Vascular aspect of glomerulus.* Kidney of human fetus, 3 months (× 590).

During septation of the cloaca, the urogenital sinus is formed. At the same time, the distal parts of the two Wolffian ducts, on the posterior side of the sinus, undergo a complex development.

In the urogenital sinus, two regions can be distinguished, according to the opening of the Wolffian ducts:

— the upper region is the **urinary zone,** which will be studied in this section;

— the lower region, or **genital zone,** will be studied with the genital system.

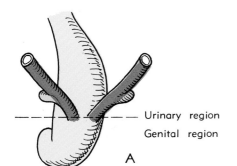

Urinary region
Genital region

A

Towards the end of the 5th week, each Wolffian duct forms a diverticulum: *the ureteric bud* (fig. 1 A).

The portion of the Wolffian duct between the beginning of the ureteric bud and the posterior wall of the urogenital sinus enlarges into a large ampulla or *horn of the urogenital sinus*. Into it, the ureter and the Wolffian duct open side by side (fig. 1 B).

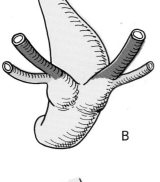

B

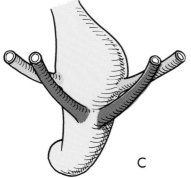

C

At 7 weeks, selective development of the posterior wall of the urogenital sinus engulfs the two horns. The ureters open separately and directly in the urogenital sinus, just outside the Wolffian ducts (fig. 1 C).

At 8 weeks, the posterior wall of the urogenital sinus continues to develop causing the orifices of the ureters to move further cranially and laterally, while the Wolffian ducts remain fixed. Modelling of the urogenital sinus causes the ureters to open into the urinary bladder and the Wolffian ducts into the urethra. The portion of the urogenital sinus wall between the openings of the ureters and the Wolffian ducts takes on a triangular form. This is the *trigonal vesicle* of mesonephric origin. It is generally thought that a temporary membrane exists at the end of the ureter (fig. 1 D).

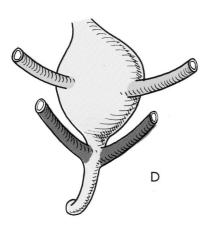

D

Fig. 1. — *Development of urogenital sinus.* Posterior views.

The allantois is progressively obliterated and forms the urachus, a fibrous cord which connects the bladder to the umbilicus.

OF UROGENITAL SINUS

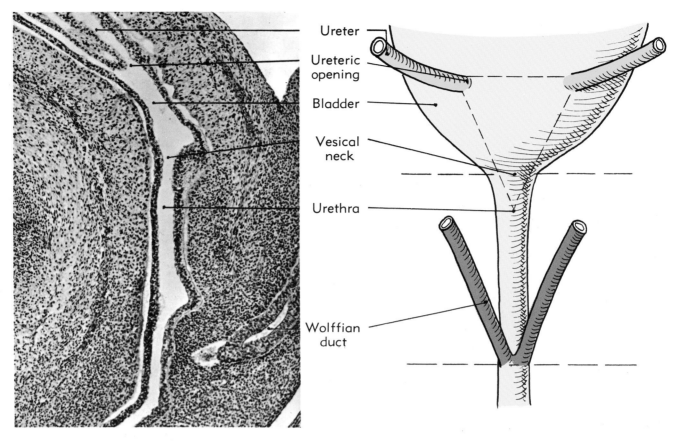

Fig. 2. — *Urogenital sinus.*

Sagittal paramedian section.
Human fetus, 2 1/4 months (× 80).

Fig. 1, E. — *Urinary zone
of urogenital sinus : the trigonal vesicle.*

Development of the urinary part of the urogenital sinus according to sex.

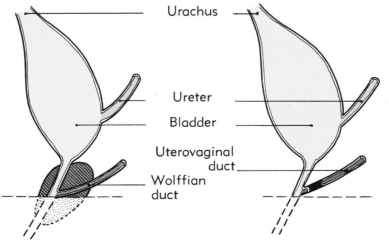

IN THE MALE

The prostate develops on both sides of the termination of the Wolffian ducts, by budding of the posterior wall of the urogenital sinus at the end of the 3rd month.

The urogenital sinus gives rise to the bladder and the upper part of the prostatic urethra.

IN THE FEMALE

Shown here is the median Müllerian uterovaginal duct, situated between the Wolffian ducts. The diagram shows the appearance of this structure after regression of the Wolffian ducts.

The urogenital sinus gives rise to the bladder and the entire urethra.

Fig. 3.

Disturbances of renal development give rise to many anomalies. In addition to hypoplasia, aplasia, and agenesis, modifications of shape and of position may be observed.

Morphologically, anomalies involving the excretory part, or the collecting portion, or both, may be distinguished.

I. — HORSESHOE KIDNEY

During migration from the sacral region, the two metanephric blastemas can come in contact with each other at one end (most often the lower pole).

They remain fused on the median line.

The ureters, which pass in front of the zone of fusion of the kidneys, are not malformed.

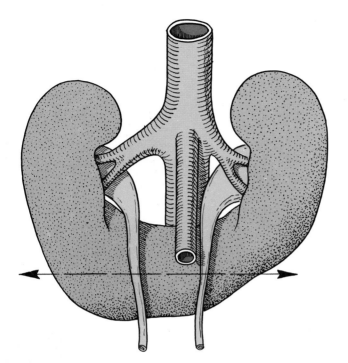

Fig. 1. — *Horseshoe kidney (classic form).* The arrow shows the plane of section of the photomicrograph below.

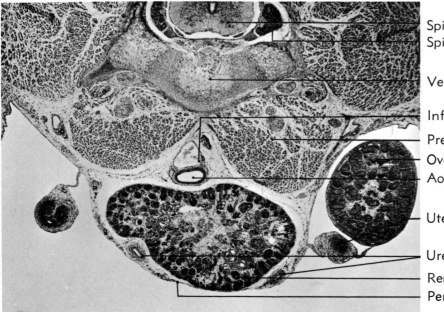

Spinal cord
Spinal ganglion

Vertebral body

Inferior vena cava
Prevertebral muscles
Ovary
Aorta

Uterine horn

Ureters
Renal parenchyma
Peritoneum

Fig. 2. — *Horseshoe kidney, sectioned near its lower pole.* Cross section. Abdomen of newborn rat (× 30).

URINARY SYSTEM

II. — *POLYCYSTIC KIDNEY*

Polycystic kidney is caused by defective junction between the portion which is of metanephric origin and the derivatives of the ureteric bud.

Because of the absence of a connection between the collecting and excretory portions of the tubules, urine cannot be evacuated (*arrow in fig. 3*).

Pressure increases in the glomerulo-tubular system and finally causes distension. Cystic degeneration occurs, and the kidney rapidly loses all functional ability.

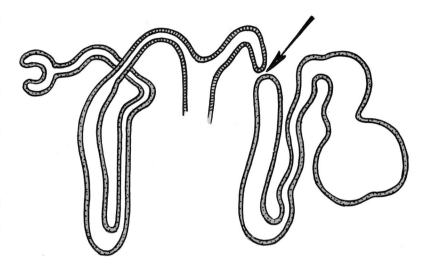

Fig. 3. — *Formation of polycystic kidney.*

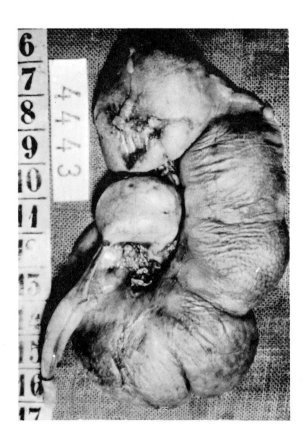

Fig. 4. — *Polycystic kidney :* gross morphology.

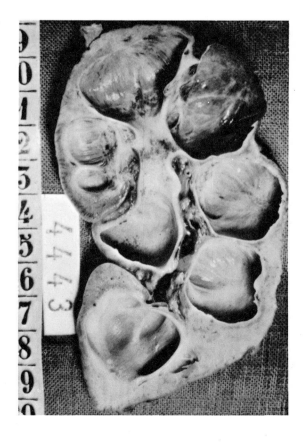

Fig. 5. — *Polycystic kidney :* section.

III. — RENAL DUPLICATIONS

Renal duplications are probably rather frequent, but many remain completely latent without any effect on urinary function.

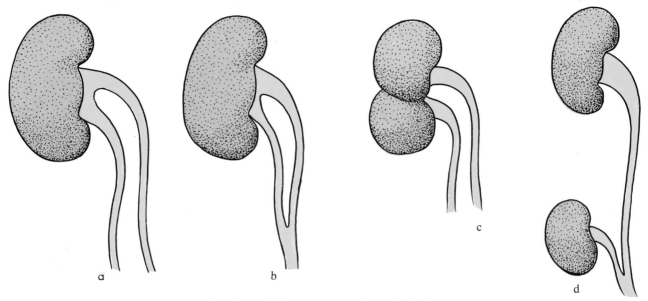

Fig. 1. — *Different types of renal duplication.*

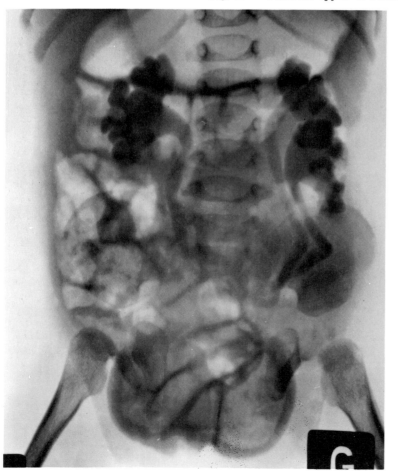

Fig. 2. — *Intravenous urography of renal duplication.*

The more or less precocious division of the ureteric bud into two branches can bring about formation of:

— *a)* **complete double ureter;**
— *b)* **partial double ureter;**
— *c)* **double kidney,** where division also involves the blastema.

In certain cases, one of the two ureters remains very short, and the second kidney remains low. This condition is no longer a double kidney, but a **supernumerary kidney** (*d*).

IV. — CONGENITAL HYDRONEPHROSES

Congenital hydronephroses involve dilatation of the renal pelvis and the calyces, bringing about reduced thickness of the cortex.

This anomaly results from a problem of urine elimination by the ureter, in turn provoked by a **high ureteral obstruction:**

— fusion of the pyeloureteral junction (normal in the embryo, but should not persist);

— compression by an aberrant vessel (inferior polar artery), or because of an abnormal path (ureter behind vena cava);

— mucosal narrowing;

— anomaly of development of ureteric bud, leading to high insertion of the ureter on the pelvis.

In the case of **low ureteral obstruction** (abnormal persistence of the ureteral membrane), the ureter itself is also dilated; this is *ureterohydronephrosis.*

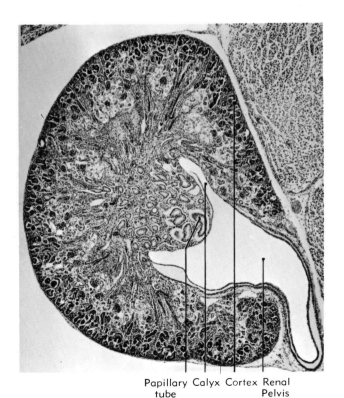

Papillary   Calyx   Cortex   Renal
tube   Pelvis

Fig. 3. — *Normal kidney.*

Newborn rat ($\times$ 37).

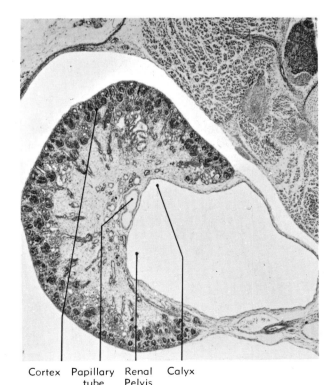

Cortex   Papillary   Renal   Calyx
tube   Pelvis

Fig. 4. — *Hydronephrotic kidney.*

Newborn rat ($\times$ 37).

COMPARATIVE VIEWS OF A NORMAL KIDNEY AND A HYDRONEPHROTIC KIDNEY.
Thinning of the cortex, distension of the pelvis and the calyces,
and dilation of the papillary ducts are seen.

PRIMORDIAL GERM CELLS

The genital glands, or gonads, testis and ovary, are formed from two types of cells:

— *reproductive germinal cells,* the primordial germ cells;

— *nutrient supporting cells,* Sertoli cells for the testis, follicular cells for the ovary.

This duality is explained by the different embryological origin of these elements.

Primordial germ cells. — The primordial germ cells are large cells, 25 to 30 µ, with granular cytoplasm, rich in lipids, and containing a large attraction sphere, or idiozome (two centrioles surrounded by Golgi apparatus) (fig. 1).

Human primordial germ cells are discernable at about 21 days, in the umbilical vesicle wall, near the allantois (fig. 2 and 3).

They thus appear at some distance from their definitive location.

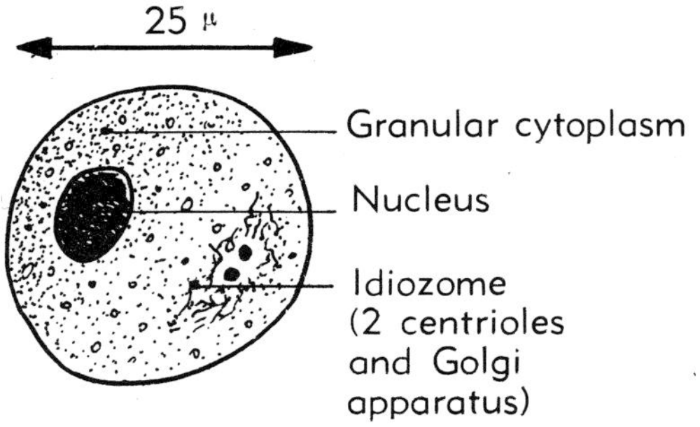

25 µ

Granular cytoplasm

Nucleus

Idiozome
(2 centrioles
and Golgi
apparatus)

Fig. 1. — *The primordial germ cell.*

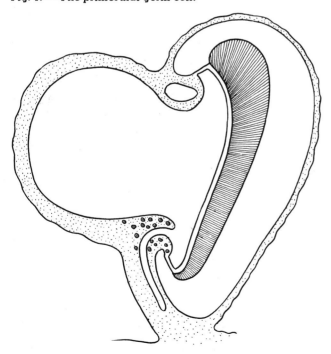

Fig. 2. — ***Origin of primordial germ cells.*** Sagittal section of human embryo of 21 days. Primordial germ cells (in red) appear along the allantois.

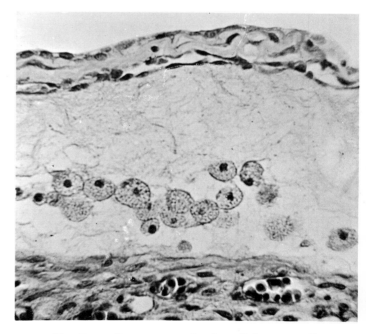

Fig. 3. — ***Appearance of primordial germ cells.*** Human embryo of 28 days (× 600).

SYSTEM

GONADAL PRIMORDIUM

During the 5th week, the primordial germ cells migrate in the dorsal mesentery and reach the lumbar region. The coelomic epithelium lining the anterior internal side of the Wolffian body thickens, forming the genital ridge: this structure provides the nutrient supporting cells of the gonad.

In the 6th week, the primordial germ cells invade the genital ridges. The ridges proliferate, forming the *primitive sexual cords,* which will become the seminiferous tubules in the male and the medullary cords in the female.

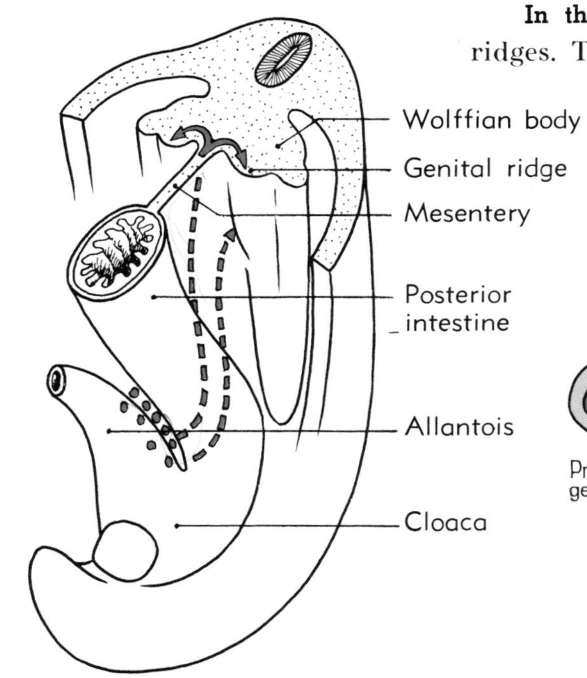

— Wolffian body

— Genital ridge

— Mesentery

— Posterior intestine

— Allantois

— Cloaca

Migration

Coelomic epithelium

Primordial germ cell

Proliferation

Fig. 4. — *Migration of primordial germ cells.*

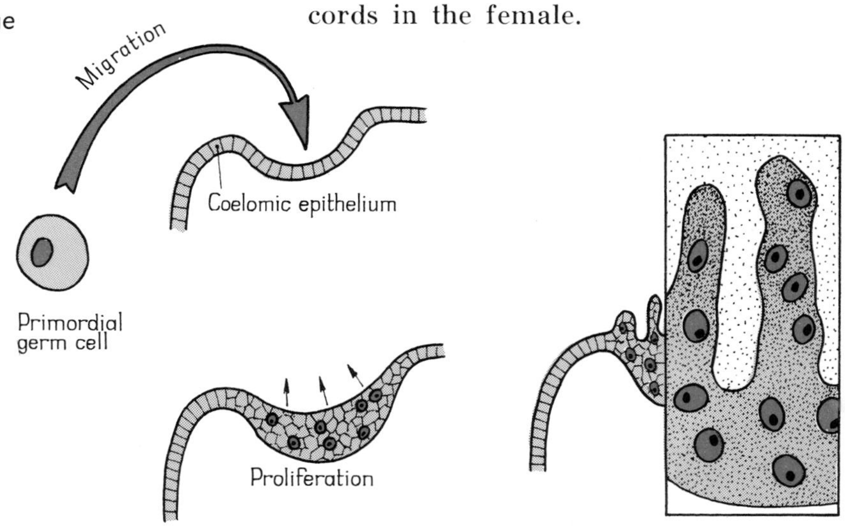

Fig. 6. — *Diagram illustrating migration of primordial germ cells.*

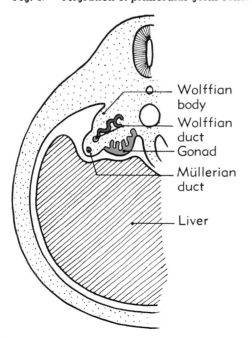

— Wolffian body

— Wolffian duct

— Gonad

— Müllerian duct

— Liver

Fig. 5. — *Indifferent gonad at time of appearance of primitive sex cords.*

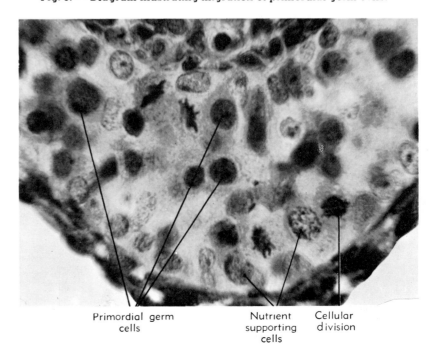

Primordial germ cells

Nutrient supporting cells

Cellular division

Fig. 7. — *Cellular duality of the gonad.*
15-day rat embryo ($\times$ 1,000).

INDIFFERENT GONAD

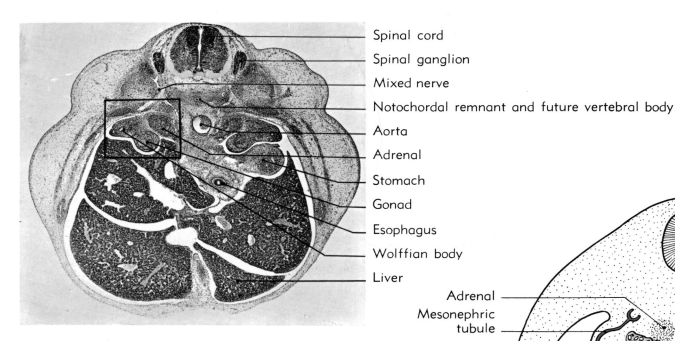

Spinal cord
Spinal ganglion
Mixed nerve
Notochordal remnant and future vertebral body
Aorta
Adrenal
Stomach
Gonad
Esophagus
Wolffian body
Liver

Fig. 1. — *Indifferent gonad in relation to body.*
Cross section of abdomen of rat embryo,
15 days (× 24).

The primitive sex cords continue to proliferate actively, and anastamose deep in the mesenchyme, producing a complex network or ***rete*** (fig. 3).

These structures bulge under the coelomic epithelium, on the anterointernal side of the Wolffian body (fig. 1 and 2).

Adrenal
Mesonephric tubule

Wolffian duct

Müllerian duct

Primitive sex cords

Gonad   Liver

Fig. 3. — *Indifferent gonad at time of formation of rete.*

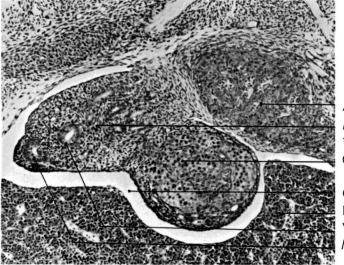

Adrenal
Mesonephric tubule
Gonad

Coelomic cavity
Liver
Wolffian duct
Müllerian duct

Fig. 2. — *Detail of gonadal primordium.*
Same preparation as figure 1 (× 120).

FIRST UROGENITAL CONNECTIONS

The rete anastomoses with the adjacent part of the mesonephric proximal convoluted tubules, thus establishing the *first urogenital connections.*

Until the end of the 6th week, the gonad has the same morphological appearance in both sexes; *it is undifferentiated.*

Towards the end of the 2nd month the Wolffian body begins to regress, the glomeruli disappear, and only the mesonephric tubules remain linked with the genital gland.

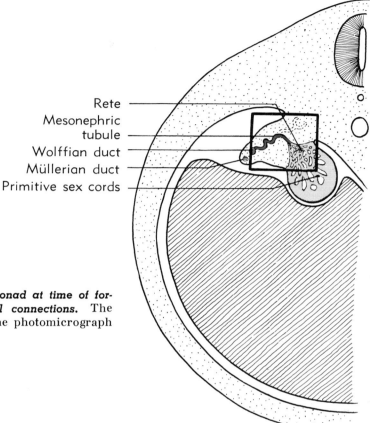

Rete
Mesonephric tubule
Wolffian duct
Müllerian duct
Primitive sex cords

Fig. 4. — *Undifferentiated gonad at time of formation of first urogenital connections.* The box shows the area of the photomicrograph in figure 5 below.

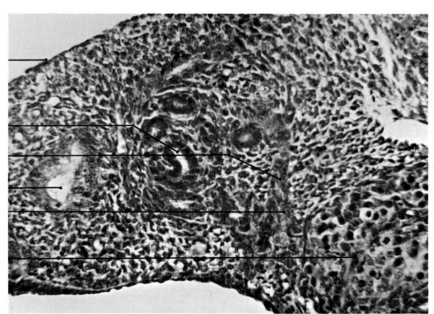

Coelomic epithelium

Mesonephric tubule

Urogenital connection

Wolffian duct

Rete

Primitive sex cords

Fig. 5. — *First urogenital connections.*
Cross section passing through gonad and Wolffian body.
Rat embryo, 15 days (× 300).

Until the 7th week of development, the genital tracts have the same appearance in both male and female embryos: they consist of the *two Wolffian ducts* and the *two Müllerian ducts*.

— Development of the **Wolffian ducts** has been studied in the chapter on the urinary system.

— In the 10 mm embryo, the **Müllerian ducts** form from an invagination of coelomic epithelium opposite the cranial end of each Wolffian duct.

An epithelial bud is formed which penetrates the mesenchyme and progresses caudally, along the Wolffian duct. The bud hollows out at the same time it grows, and becomes an open duct in the coelomic cavity.

At the lower pole of the Wolffian body, the Müllerian duct crosses in front of the Wolffian duct and thereafter runs alongside it. It inflects toward the median line and joins the Müllerian duct from the opposite side. The terminal part of the ducts fuse, forming a small single median duct which ends blind at the posterior side of the urogenital sinus. This is the Müllerian tubercle, between the orifices of the Wolffian ducts.

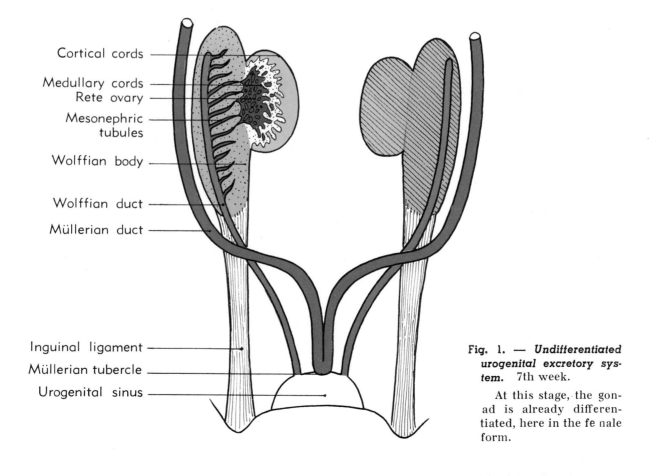

Cortical cords
Medullary cords
Rete ovary
Mesonephric tubules
Wolffian body
Wolffian duct
Müllerian duct
Inguinal ligament
Müllerian tubercle
Urogenital sinus

Fig. 1. — *Undifferentiated urogenital excretory system.* 7th week.

At this stage, the gonad is already differentiated, here in the female form.

GENITAL TRACTS

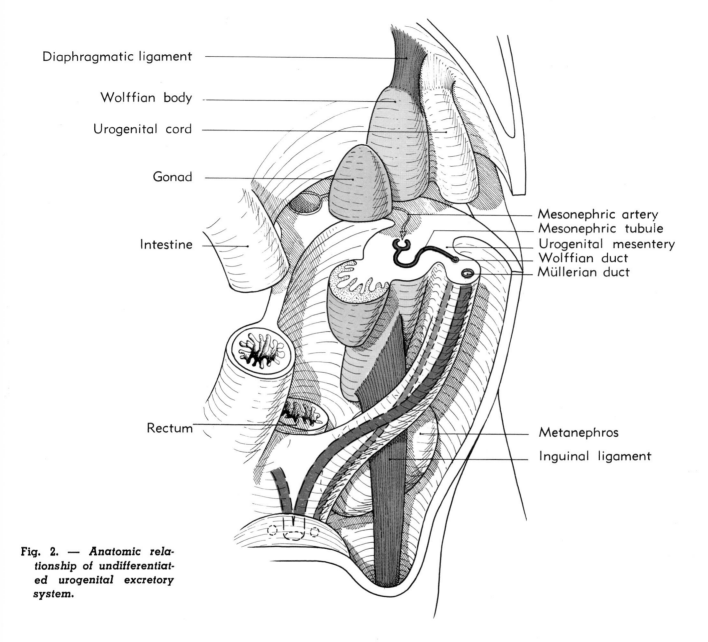

Diaphragmatic ligament

Wolffian body

Urogenital cord

Gonad

Intestine

Rectum

Mesonephric artery
Mesonephric tubule
Urogenital mesentery
Wolffian duct
Müllerian duct

Metanephros

Inguinal ligament

Fig. 2. — Anatomic relationship of undifferentiated urogenital excretory system.

The Wolffian and Müllerian ducts are situated in the **urogenital cord** attached to the anterior external edge of the Wolffian body by the **urogenital mesentery;** this in turn attaches the urogenital cord to the body wall, below the Wolffian body.

The two urogenital mesenteries, right and left, join below on the median line.

Throughout its length, the Wolffian body is attached to the abdominal wall by the **Wolffian mesentery.** Above the Wolffian body, the urogenital mesentery and the Wolffian mesentery extend upward and form the **diaphragmatic ligament.**

The lower pole of the Wolffian body is attached at the inguinal region by the **inguinal ligament.**

TESTICULAR DIFFERENTIATION

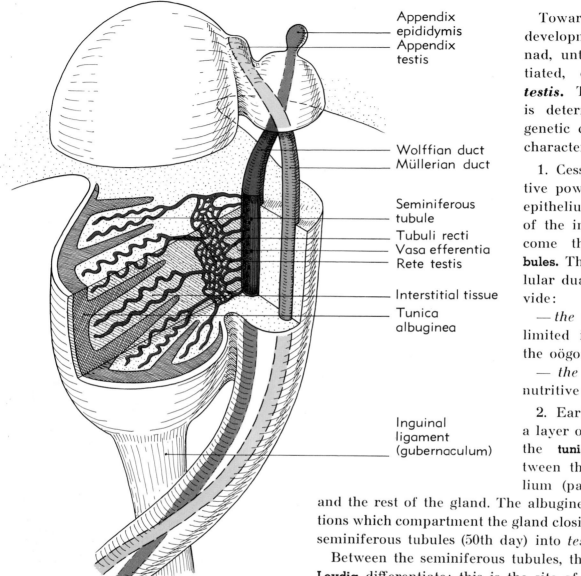

Appendix
epididymis
Appendix
testis

Wolffian duct
Müllerian duct

Seminiferous
tubule
Tubuli recti
Vasa efferentia
Rete testis

Interstitial tissue
Tunica
albuginea

Inguinal
ligament
(gubernaculum)

*Fig. 1. — Testicular differentiation
at time of regression of the Wolffian body.*

Towards the 7th week of development, the male gonad, until then undifferentiated, develops into the **testis.** This differentiation is determined by the XY genetic constitution, and is characterized by:

1. Cessation of proliferative power of the coelomic epithelium: the sex cords of the indifferent stage become the **seminiferous tubules.** These, with their cellular duality of origin, provide:

— *the spermatogonia,* unlimited in number (unlike the oögonia), and

— *the Sertoli cells,* or nutritive supporting cells.

2. Early interposition of a layer of connective tissue, the **tunica albuginea,** between the coelomic epithelium (parietal peritoneum) and the rest of the gland. The albuginea puts forth partitions which compartment the gland closing off the rolled-up seminiferous tubules (50th day) into *testis cords.*

Between the seminiferous tubules, the **interstitial cells of Leydig** differentiate; this is the site of elaboration of the androgenic hormones which mold differentiation of the tract and the external genital organs. The Leydig, or interstitial cells of the testis, reach their maximum development between 3 1/2 and 4 months.

3. The deep portion of the seminiferous tubules of each testis cord narrows to form the **tubulus rectus.** The tubuli recti converge in the **rete testis.**

The Sertoli cells, the tubuli recti, and the rete testis all arise from coelomic epithelium.

4. After regression of the Wolffian body, part of the mesonephric tubules participates in formation of the excretory tracts of the testis, forming the **vasa efferentia.**

The vasa efferentia eventually open into the segment adjacent to the Wolffian duct which becomes the **epididymis.**

The vasa efferentia and the epididymis are of mesonephric origin.

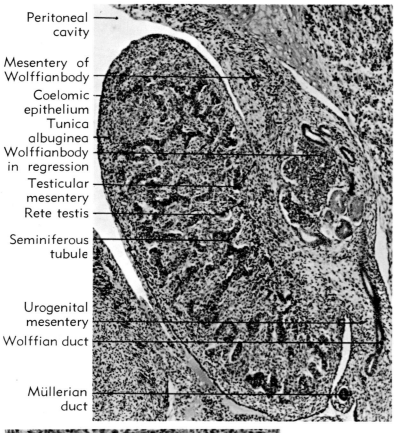

Peritoneal cavity

Mesentery of Wolffian body

Coelomic epithelium
Tunica albuginea

Wolffian body in regression

Testicular mesentery

Rete testis

Seminiferous tubule

Urogenital mesentery

Wolffian duct

Müllerian duct

Fig. 2 *(opposite).* — *Differentiating testis.* Longitudinal section. Fetus, 2 months (× 75).

Fig. 3 *(below at left).* — *Differentiating testis.* Fetus 3 1/2 months (× 145). Light-colored spermatogonia can be distinguished in the seminiferous tubules.

Fig. 4 *(below).* — *Differentiated testis.* Structure of whole testis. Longitudinal section. Fetus, 3 1/2 months (× 30).

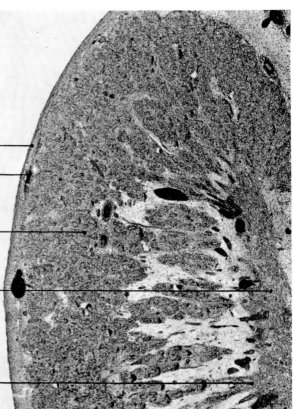

Peritoneum

Tunica albuginea

Seminiferous tubules

Rete testis

Tubuli recti

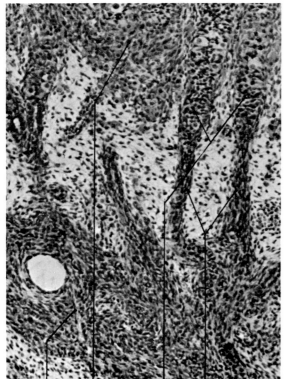

Rete testis   Leydig   Seminiferous tubule   Tubuli recti

I. — UPPER PORTION

Male differentiation of the urogenital excretory system is due to the action of androgenic fetal hormones. This effect begins at the end of the 2nd month and is seen in the regression of Müllerian structures, and development and differentiation of Wolffian structures.

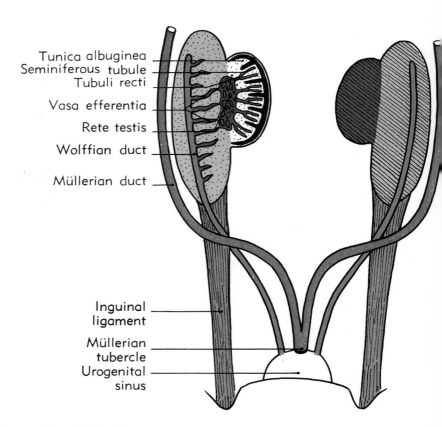

Tunica albuginea
Seminiferous tubule
Tubuli recti
Vasa efferentia
Rete testis
Wolffian duct
Müllerian duct

Inguinal ligament
Müllerian tubercle
Urogenital sinus

Fig. 1. — *Urogenital excretory system during differentiation of the male.*

Appendix epididymis
Appendix testis
Tunica albuginea
Vasa efferentia
Prolongation of tunica albuginea
Seminiferous tubule
Rete testis
Wolffian duct
Epididymis
Gubernaculum testis

Müllerian duct
Ductus deferens

Seminal vesicle

Ejaculatory duct
Utriculus prostaticus

Verumontanum

Fig. 2.

Differentiated male urogenital excretory system.

After regression of the Wolffian body, the inguinal ligament inserts at the inferior pole of the testis above, and in the inguinal region below. This forms the *gubernaculum testis.* The diaphragmatic ligament disappears.

Both Müllerian ducts regress completely by the 11th week. The *appendix testis,* however, persists at the superior pole of each testis. Below, the *utriculus prostaticus,* opening on the midline, persists from the early joining of the Müllerian ducts. This is placed on the posterior side of the urogenital sinus, between the Wolffian ducts (fig. 2).

MALE GENITAL TRACTS

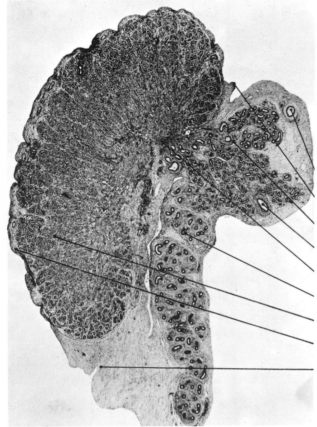

Head of epididymis
(upper section)
Appendix testis

Mass of vasa
efferentia
Head of epididymis
(lower section)
Rete testis

Epididymis,
convoluted
Seminiferous tubules

Tunica albuginea

Gubernaculum testis

Fig. 3. — *Gubernaculum testis, vasa efferentia, epididymis.* Longitudinal section of testis. Fetus, 4 months (× 17).

The **two Wolffian ducts** persist and develop in a complex way:

— At the most cranial portion on the end of the epididymis, the *appendix epididymis* is formed.

— The segment of the Wolffian duct opposite the testis forms the *epididymis*. Its cranial portion is connected to the vasa efferentia. Below the cranial end, the epididymis is highly convoluted and descends along the testis receiving several mesonephric tubules not connected with the rete testis: the *ducts of Haller*. Below, certain isolated mesonephric tubules form the *paradidymis*.

— Below the testis, the Wolffian duct becomes the *ductus deferens*.

— Just before it joins the posterior side of the urogenital sinus, each ductus deferens swells, forming an ampulla and a hollow diverticulum, *the seminal vesicle*.

— Caudally, the ductus deferens becomes the *ejaculatory duct*. Between the two ejaculatory ducts is the *utriculus prostaticus*.

— The ejaculatory ducts and the utriculus prostaticus open on the posterior side of the urogenital sinus, at the level of the *verumontanum*.

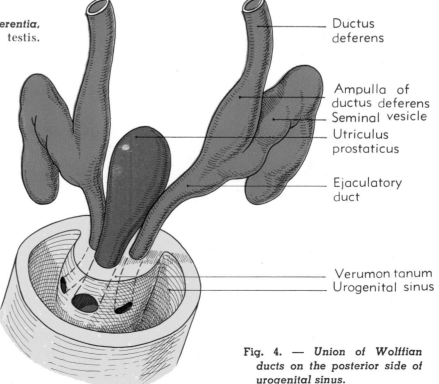

Ductus
deferens

Ampulla of
ductus deferens
Seminal vesicle
Utriculus
prostaticus

Ejaculatory
duct

Verumontanum
Urogenital sinus

Fig. 4. — *Union of Wolffian ducts on the posterior side of urogenital sinus.*

The lower portion of the male genital tract is the section of the urogenital sinus caudal to the union of the Wolffian ducts. It consists of two parts:

— a vertical *pelvic segment;*

— a horizontal *phallic segment* in the genital tubercle. After resorption of the urogenital membrane it is open to the exterior (fig. 2).

From the third month, these two segments of the urogenital sinus undergo a complex reorganization related to secretion of androgenic hormones.

Only the **pelvic segment** will be studied here; the phallic segment will be studied with the external genital organs.

During the 3rd month, the epithelial buds begin to detach themselves from the posterior side of the urogenital sinus on both sides of the verumontanum. They penetrate the adjacent mesenchyme and form the **prostate,** which is well differentiated at 4 months.

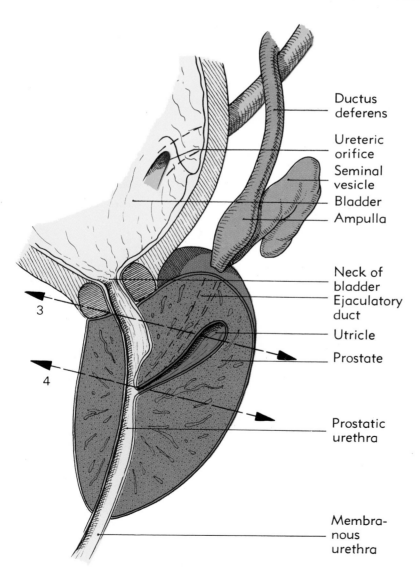

Ductus deferens

Ureteric orifice

Seminal vesicle

Bladder

Ampulla

Neck of bladder

Ejaculatory duct

Utricle

Prostate

Prostatic urethra

Membranous urethra

3

4

The prostate eventually encloses the ejaculatory ducts and the utriculus prostaticus. It completely surrounds an area of the urogenital sinus, the **prostatic urethra.**

The prostatic urethra is formed of:

— a caudal half, caudal to the verumontanum, which belongs to the urinary region of the urogenital sinus, caudal to the bladder;

— a caudal half, caudal of the verumontanum, the cranial part of the pelvic segment of the urogenital sinus.

The rest of the pelvic segment forms the **membranous urethra,** which is continuous with the phallic segment.

Fig. 1. — *Prostatic urethra and membranous urethra.* Right half of prostate. (Note the 2 planes of section corresponding to figures 3 and 4).

MALE GENITAL TRACT

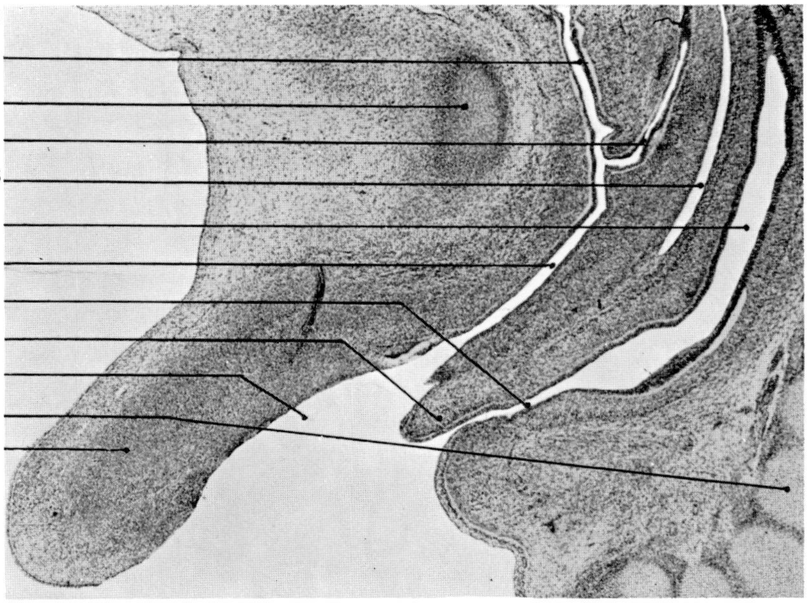

Urinary portion of urogenital sinus

Symphysis pubis

Wolffian duct

Rectouterine pouch of Douglas

Rectum

Pelvic segment of urogenital sinus

Anal canal

Perineum

Urogenital groove

Vertebral column

Penile genital tubercle

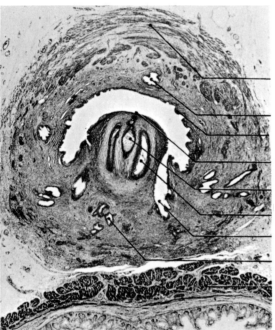

Smooth muscles

Prostatic gland

Urethral glands

Bulge of verumontanum in the prostatic urethra

Prostatic utricle

Ejaculatory duct

Union of prostatic ducts

Prostatic gland

Rectal muscle

Rectal lumen

Fig. 2. — *Genital portion of male urogenital sinus after resorption of urogenital membrane.* Median sagittal section. Fetus in the 10th week (× 30).

Fig. 3. — *Verumontanum.* Transverse section. Fetus of 4 months (× 20). (*See arrow 4, fig. 1.*)

Smooth muscle of sphincter in neck of bladder

Prostatic urethra (cranial half)

Prostatic utricle

Prostatic gland

Ejaculatory duct

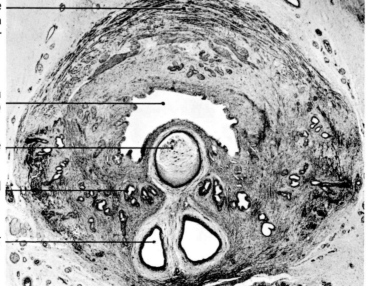

Fig. 4. — *Prostate.* Transverse section. Fetus of 4 months (× 20). (*See arrow 3, fig. 1.*)

Development of the external male genital organs is evident beginning the 3rd month. This differentiation is related to the action of androgens.

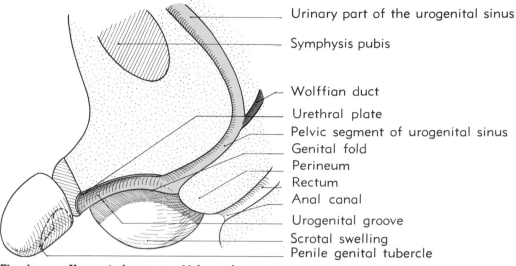

— Urinary part of the urogenital sinus
— Symphysis pubis

— Wolffian duct
— Urethral plate
— Pelvic segment of urogenital sinus
— Genital fold
— Perineum
— Rectum
— Anal canal
— Urogenital groove
— Scrotal swelling
— Penile genital tubercle

Fig. 1 a. — Urogenital groove : 11th week.

Urinary part of
urogenital sinus
Symphysis pubis
Wolffian duct
Pelvic segment of
urogenital sinus
Rectum
Anal canal
Perineum
Urogenital groove
Urethral plate
Penile genital tubercle

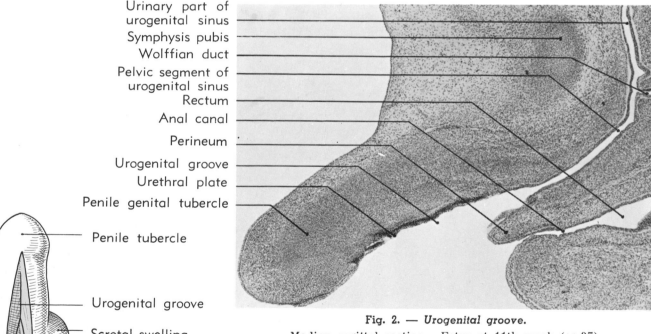

Fig. 2. — Urogenital groove.
Median sagittal section.   Fetus at 11th week ($\times$ 37).

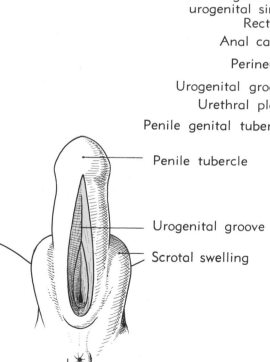

Penile tubercle

Urogenital groove

Scrotal swelling

*Fig. 1 b. — Urogenital groove
seen from below : 11th week.*

Beginning in the 11th week, the genital tubercle elongates, forming the future **penis.**

It carries with it the genital folds surrounding the phallic segment of the urogenital sinus. This elongates on the dorsal side of the penis and forms the **urogenital groove.**

At the base of this groove the entoderm thickens into a **urethral plate.**

The posterior part of the genital swellings thickens and forms the **scrotal swellings.**

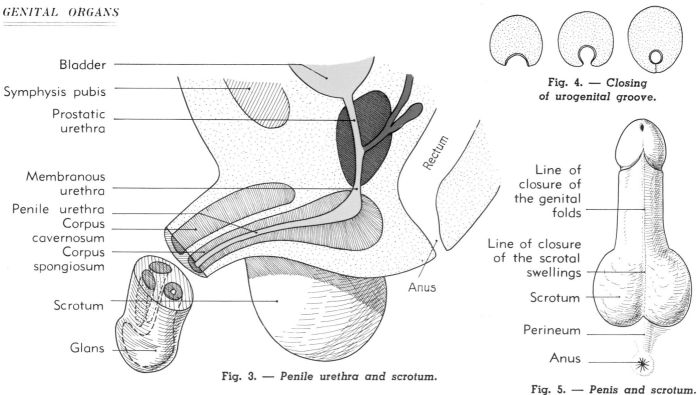

Bladder

Symphysis pubis

Prostatic urethra

Membranous urethra

Penile urethra
Corpus cavernosum
Corpus spongiosum

Scrotum

Glans

Rectum

Anus

Fig. 3. — *Penile urethra and scrotum.*

Fig. 4. — *Closing of urogenital groove.*

Line of closure of the genital folds

Line of closure of the scrotal swellings

Scrotum

Perineum

Anus

Fig. 5. — *Penis and scrotum.*

At about 3 months, the genital folds circumscribing the median urogenital groove fuse, changing the groove into a duct: **the penile urethra** (fig. 4).

The penile urethra ends blindly just before the end of the penis. It is surrounded by a mass of erectile tissue of mesenchymal origin: *the corpus spongiosum.* The erectile tissue of the glans forms the protuberant end of the penis.

Within the shaft of the penis, the paired *corpora cavernosa* complete the erectile system (fig. 3 and 6).

The scrotal swellings fuse on the median line and form the **scrotum.**

Penis and scrotum carry the signs of their formation through closure of the urogenital groove in the *median raphe* (fig. 5).

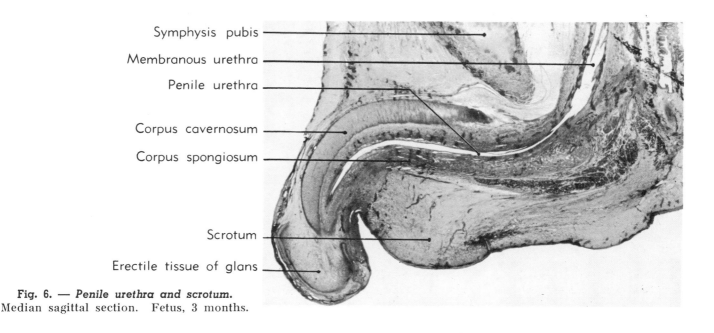

Symphysis pubis

Membranous urethra

Penile urethra

Corpus cavernosum

Corpus spongiosum

Scrotum

Erectile tissue of glans

Fig. 6. — *Penile urethra and scrotum.*
Median sagittal section. Fetus, 3 months.

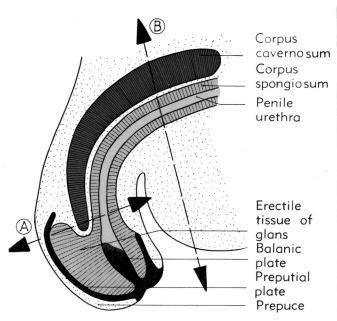

Corpus cavernosum
Corpus spongiosum
Penile urethra

Erectile tissue of glans
Balanic plate
Preputial plate
Prepuce

Fig. 1. — *Glandular and preputial epithelial plates.*

During the 4th month, the epithelial covering of the end of the penis forms 2 invaginations.

— One forms a solid epithelial cord; this is the **glandular epithelial plate** which rapidly

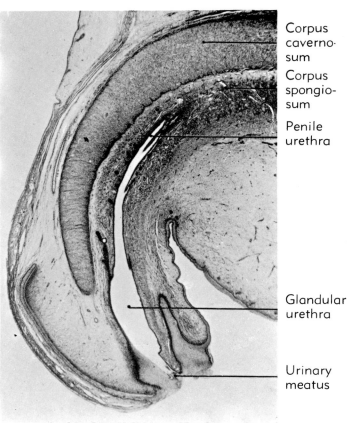

Corpus cavernosum
Corpus spongiosum
Penile urethra

Glandular urethra

Urinary meatus

Fig. 2. — *Glandular urethra.*
Sagittal section. Fetus of 4 months (× 20).

hollows out to form the **glandular urethra** opening at the urinary meatus.
— The other is circular: this is the **preputial epithelial plate;** cleavage of this plate before birth separates the glans from the prepuce.

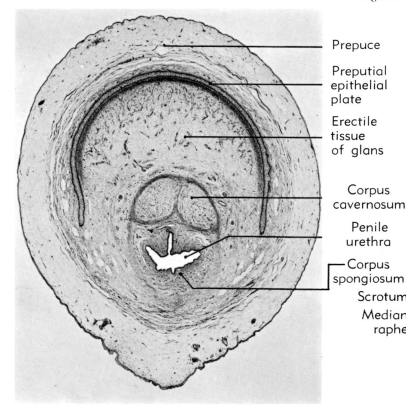

Prepuce

Preputial epithelial plate

Erectile tissue of glans

Corpus cavernosum

Corpus spongiosum

Fig. 3. — *Erectile system at level of glans.*
Plane of section A of fig. 1. Fetus of 4 months (× 20).

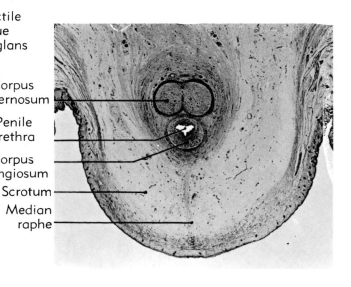

Corpus cavernosum

Penile urethra

Corpus spongiosum
Scrotum
Median raphe

Fig. 4. – *Erectile system in relation to scrotum.*
Plane of section B of figure 1. Fetus of 4 months (× 10).

IV. — TESTICULAR MIGRATION

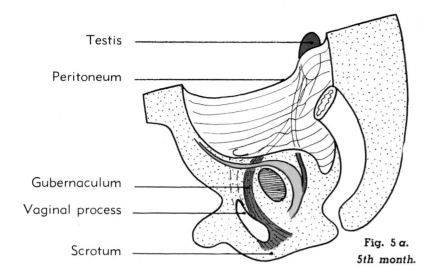

Testis
Peritoneum
Gubernaculum
Vaginal process
Scrotum

Fig. 5 a.
5th month.

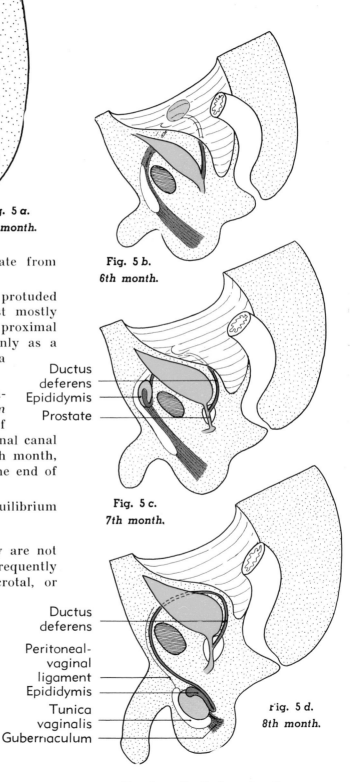

Fig. 5 b.
6th month.

Ductus deferens
Epididymis
Prostate

Fig. 5 c.
7th month.

Ductus deferens
Peritoneal-vaginal ligament
Epididymis
Tunica vaginalis
Gubernaculum

Fig. 5 d.
8th month.

Fig. 5. — *Testicular migration.*

Between the 3rd month and term, the testes migrate from their primitively lumbar position to the scrotum.

A bilateral prolongation of the coelomic cavity is protuded into the scrotum, the *vaginal process.* This is at first mostly open, then progressively narrowed, and finally, the proximal portion is entirely obliterated. The rest then exists only as a double serous enveloppe around the testis, the tunica vaginalis.

The vaginal process is parallel with the inferior ligament of the testis which becomes the *gubernaculum testis.* The migration of the gland follows the line of this structure. The testis reaches the orifice of the inguinal canal around the 6th month, crosses the canal during the 7th month, and reaches its definitive intrascrotal position toward the end of the 8th month.

This migration is regulated by precise hormonal equilibrium in which androgens and gonadotrophins participate.

Anomalies of testicular migration are numerous. They are not necessarily related to a hormonal deficit, since they are frequently unilateral. They range from *simple ectopy* (inguinoscrotal, or inguinal) to *cryptorchism* (pelvic, iliac, or lumbar). The gland may also be in an aberrant location, crural or perineal. Cryptorchism always brings about an alteration in spermatogenesis, or, if bilateral, sterility.

Anomalies of closure of vaginal processes are also very frequent. They are sometimes, but not obligatorily, associated with problems of testicular migration. Cysts of the spermatic cord are signs of incomplete closure. A complete failure of closure may cause congenital *oblique external hernia* or so-called "communicating" *hydrocoele.*

OVARIAN DIFFERENTIATION

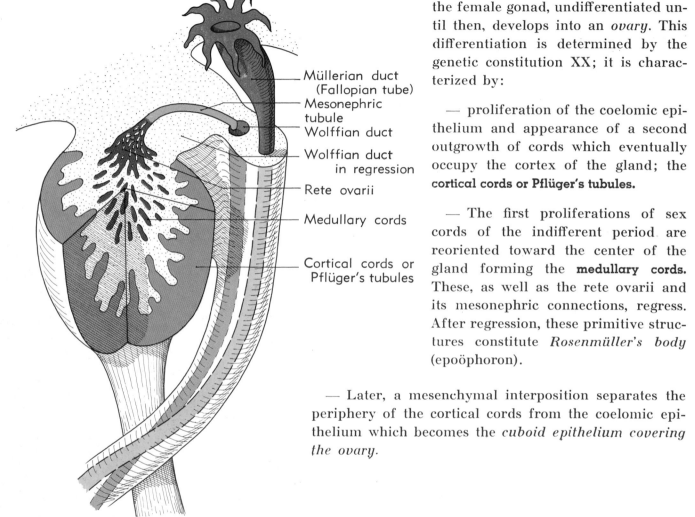

Müllerian duct
(Fallopian tube)

Mesonephric
tubule

Wolffian duct

Wolffian duct
in regression

Rete ovarii

Medullary cords

Cortical cords or
Pflüger's tubules

About the 7th week of development, the female gonad, undifferentiated until then, develops into an *ovary*. This differentiation is determined by the genetic constitution XX; it is characterized by:

— proliferation of the coelomic epithelium and appearance of a second outgrowth of cords which eventually occupy the cortex of the gland; the **cortical cords or Pflüger's tubules.**

— The first proliferations of sex cords of the indifferent period are reoriented toward the center of the gland forming the **medullary cords.** These, as well as the rete ovarii and its mesonephric connections, regress. After regression, these primitive structures constitute *Rosenmüller's body* (epoöphoron).

— Later, a mesenchymal interposition separates the periphery of the cortical cords from the coelomic epithelium which becomes the *cuboid epithelium covering the ovary.*

Fig. 1. — *Diagrammatic view of ovarian differentiation at time of regression of Wolffian body.*

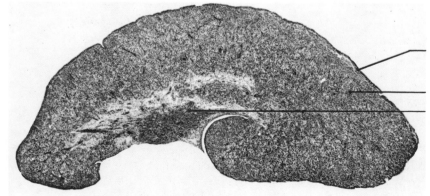

Cuboid surface epithelium

Cortical cords

Medullary cords and rete ovarii

Fig. 2. — *Cortical and medullary cords.* Longitudinal section of ovary. Fetus, 3 months ($\times$ 28).

SYSTEM

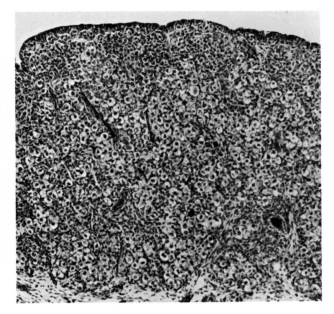

Fig. 3. — *Cortical cords before fragmentation.* The oögonia appear clear. Human fetus, 3 months (× 100).

Each oögonium is surrounded by a layer of supporting cells, **the follicular cells.**

The primordial follicles demonstrate the cellular duality of the undifferentiated gonadal primordium; they are distributed in a connective tissue stroma. Their number is limited: about 300,000 are present at birth. They contain a specific reproductive cell, the **oöcyte at the primary stage,** with 46 chromosomes (fig. 4 and 5).

Until the 5th month, the cortical cords are trabecular in appearance. Among them can be seen islets of large cells with clear cytoplasm, the **oögonia,** in the midst of **supporting nutrient cells** (originating from the coelomic epithelium).

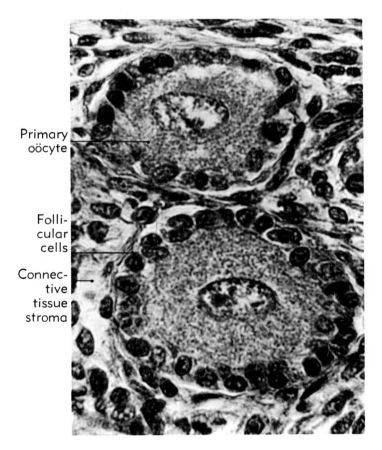

Primary oöcyte

Follicular cells

Connective tissue stroma

Fig. 4. — *Primordial follicles.* Human ovary. Fetus, 9 months (× 775).

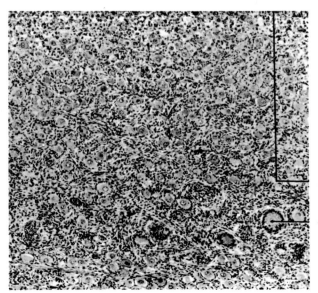

Cuboid ovarian epithelium

Primordial follicle

Fig. 5. ***The ovarian cortex at birth*** (× 75).

Of the initial stock of primordial follicles, about 300 develop between puberty and menopause to produce fertilizable ova.

Towards the 8th week, the caudal segments of the two **Müllerian ducts** fuse above their crossing of the inguinal ligament, to form the single median uterovaginal canal. The fusion begins caudally and progresses up to the future Fallopian tubes. The median septum disappears at the end of the 3rd month.

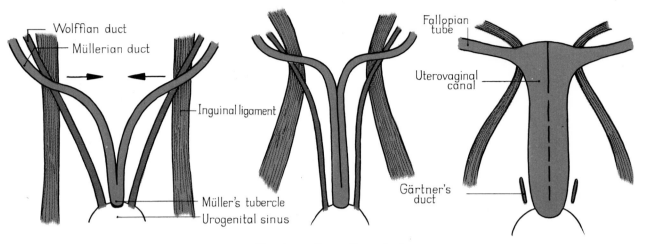

Fig. 1. — *Formation of uterus.*

The upper part of the uterovaginal canal provides the epithelium of the uterine mucosa. The uterine muscle layer, or myometrium, differentiates from the connective tissue girdle resulting from fusion of the urogenital cords. The mesenchymal covering is attached to the abdominal wall on each side by the broad ligaments, a continuation of the urogenital mesentery.

The two **Wolffian ducts** regress, persisting in the vestigial structures called *Gärtner's ducts* (fig. 1). Caudal to the Fallopian tubes, the inguinal ligament becomes the round ligament.

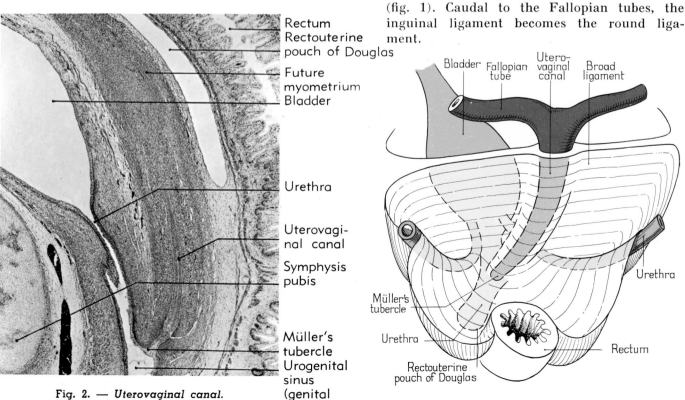

Fig. 2. — *Uterovaginal canal.*
Sagittal median section.
Fetus 2 1/2 months (× 30).

Fig. 3. — *Uterovaginal canal and broad ligament.*

FEMALE GENITAL TRACT

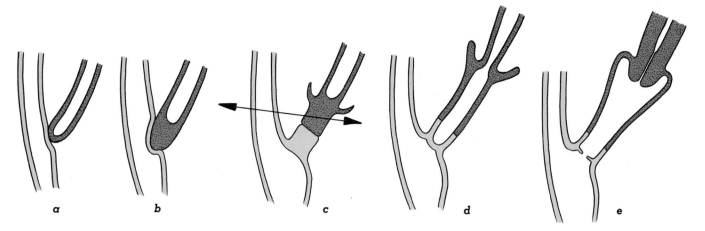

Fig. 4. — *Formation of vagina.*

a. The terminal end of the primitive uterovaginal canal touches the posterior side of the urogenital sinus and forms **Müller's tubercle.**

b. Müller's tubercle thickens and temporarily elongates the uterine cavity of the urogenital sinus.

c. The posterior wall of the urogenital sinus thickens opposite the tubercle, and with it forms the **vaginal epithelial plate.** From this, two solid evaginations encircle the caudal end of the uterine canal.

d. Canalization of the vaginal plate proceeds from cranial to caudal end, prolonging the uterovaginal canal and forming the vagina.

e. The **sinovaginal bulbs** are now seen, surrounding the cervix.

The cranial four-fifths of the vagina are thus of mesodermic origin (Müllerian ducts), and the caudal fifth of entodermal origin (urogenital sinus). The vagina remains separated from the urogenital sinus by the *hymen.*

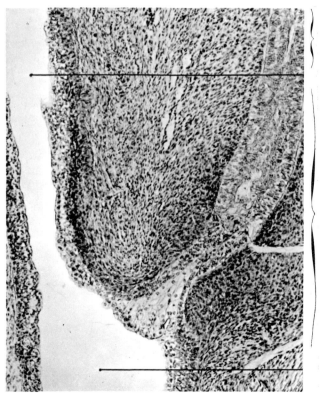

Uterus

Urethra

Vaginal epithelial plate

Urogenital sinus

Fig. 5. — *Vaginal epithelial plate.*
Median sagittal section. Fetus 2 1/2 months (×30).

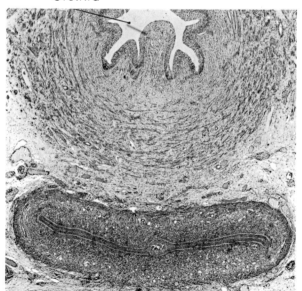

Urethra

Fig. 6. — *Vaginal epithelial plate.*
Cross section (arrow in fig. 4 *c*).
Fetus, 3 months (× 14).

After formation of the uterovaginal canal, the segment of each **Müllerian duct** which is cranial to the junction of the inguinal ligament and the urogenital cord becomes a *Fallopian tube*. The cranial orifice of the Müllerian duct, open to the peritoneal cavity, becomes the *fimbriae* of the Fallopian tube (fig. 1 and 2).

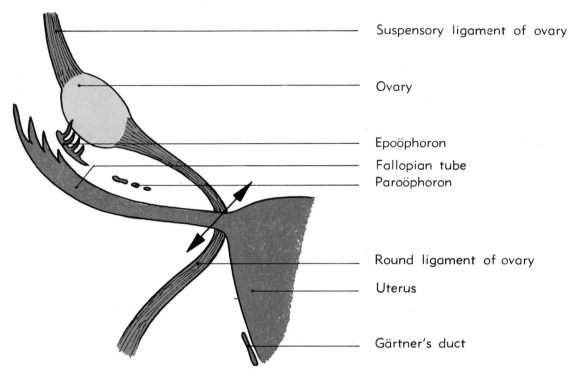

Suspensory ligament of ovary

Ovary

Epoöphoron
Fallopian tube
Paroöphoron

Round ligament of ovary

Uterus

Gärtner's duct

Fig. 1. — *Formation of Fallopian tube and Wolffian vestiges.*

The Fallopian tube moves caudally and becomes horizontal.

The Wolffian duct regresses almost completely; only a short segment connected with the mesonephric tubes adjacent to the ovary persists, the *epoöphoron* or *Rosenmüller's body*. Several mesonephric tubes caudal to the ovary form the *paroöphoron*.

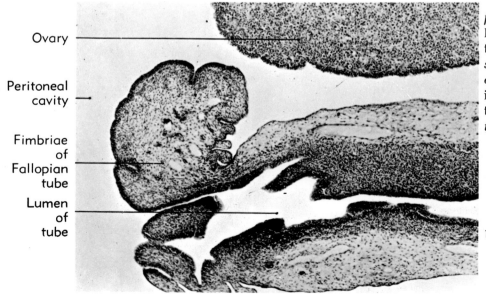

Ovary

Peritoneal cavity

Fimbriae of Fallopian tube

Lumen of tube

After regression of the *Wolffian duct*, the diaphragmatic ligament is attached directly to the ovary and becomes the *suspensory ligament of the ovary*. The inguinal ligament is also attached to the ovary; this is the *proper ligament of the ovary* (fig. 1).

Fig. 2. — *Opening of Fallopian tube in the peritoneal cavity.* Longitudinal section of Fallopian tube fimbriae. Fetus, 3 1/2 months ($\times$ 75).

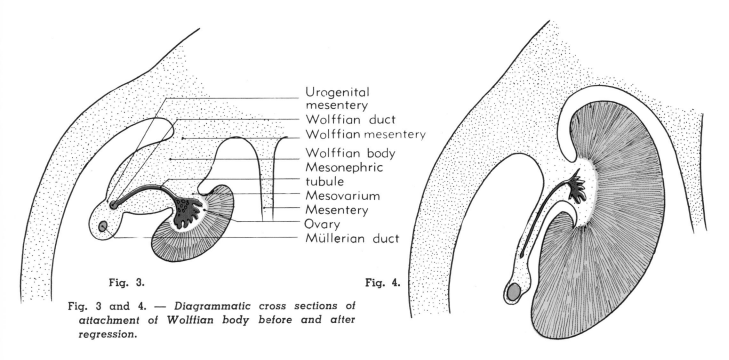

Urogenital mesentery
Wolffian duct
Wolffian mesentery
Wolffian body
Mesonephric tubule
Mesovarium
Mesentery
Ovary
Müllerian duct

Fig. 3.

Fig. 4.

Fig. 3 and 4. — *Diagrammatic cross sections of attachment of Wolffian body before and after regression.*

Beginning in the 3rd month, the Wolffian body flattens and atrophies. Only a vestige, between the urogenital and the Wolffian mesenteries, persists. These three structures together form the *mesosalpinx*, which connects the urogenital cord and the Fallopian tube to the abdominal wall. The *mesovarium* is thus attached definitively to the internal side of the mesosalpinx; this is continuous caudally with the mesometrium, forming with it the *broad ligament*.

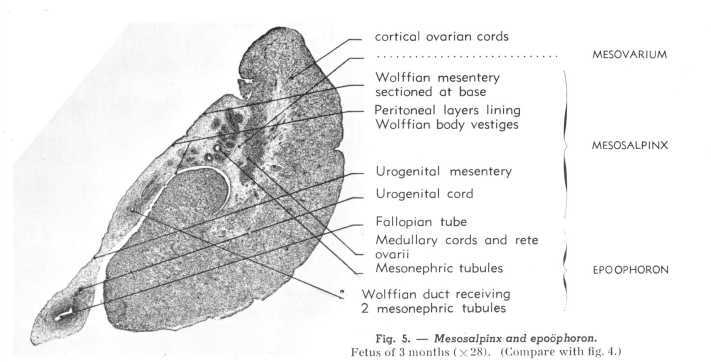

cortical ovarian cords
.... MESOVARIUM

Wolffian mesentery sectioned at base
Peritoneal layers lining Wolffian body vestiges

Urogenital mesentery
Urogenital cord

Fallopian tube
Medullary cords and rete ovarii
Mesonephric tubules

Wolffian duct receiving 2 mesonephric tubules

MESOSALPINX

EPOÖPHORON

Fig. 5. — *Mesosalpinx and epoöphoron.*
Fetus of 3 months (×28). (Compare with fig. 4.)

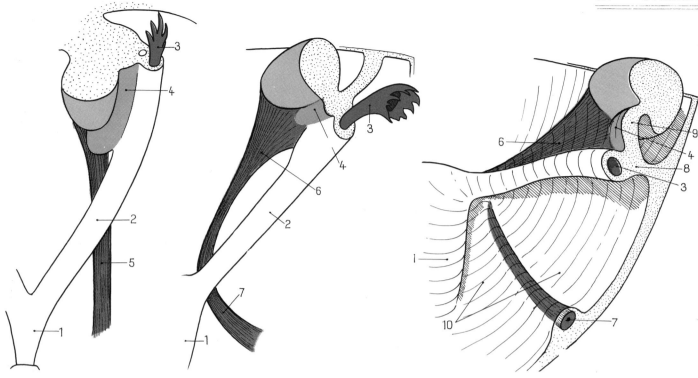

Fig. 1 a. — *Primitive vertical arrangement of urogenital cord.*

Fig. 1 b. — *Temporary location of ovary on dorsal side of regressing Wolffian body.*

Fig. 1 c. — *Beginning of posterior movement of ovary.*

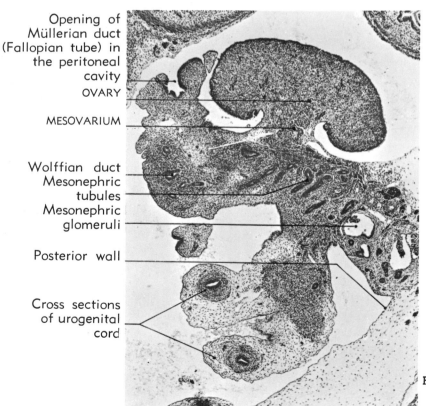

Opening of Müllerian duct (Fallopian tube) in the peritoneal cavity

OVARY

MESOVARIUM

Wolffian duct
Mesonephric tubules
Mesonephric glomeruli

Posterior wall

Cross sections of urogenital cord

Legends of figures 1 a to 1 e.

1. Uterus.
2. Urogenital cord.
3. Fallopian tube.
4. Wolffian body or its vestige.
5. Inguinal ligament.
6. Proper ligament of the ovary.
7. Round ligament of the uterus.
8. Mesosalpinx.
9. Mesovarium.
10. Broad ligament of uterus.

Fig. 2. — *Lateral sagittal section passing through regressing Wolffian body.* Fetus of 2 months ($\times$ 25).

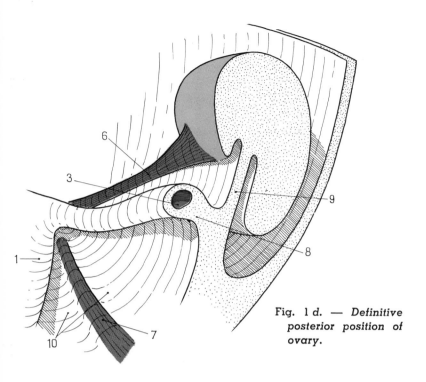

Fig. 1 d. — *Definitive posterior position of ovary.*

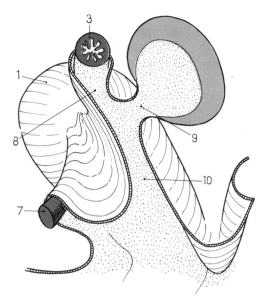

Fig. 1 e. — *Diagrammatic oblique sagittal section on the inner side of the broad ligament.*

Initially, the Fallopian tube (cranial portion of Müllerian duct) is vertical (fig. 1 *a*). During development of the uterus, it moves toward the interior of the abdominal cavity and becomes horizontal.

The ovary is located successively cranial to (fig. 1 *b*), then dorsal to (fig. 1 *c* and 1 *d*) the Fallopian tube.

The mesenteries also follow these positional changes: their definitive arrangement in the pelvis forms the **broad ligament** of the uterus with its three flanges (fig. 1 *e*) :

cranial or mesosalpinx (Fallopian tube) ;

anterior (round ligament of uterus) ;

posterior or mesovarium (proper ligament of ovary and ovary).

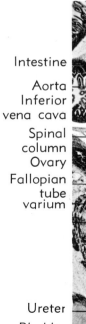

Intestine
Aorta
Inferior vena cava
Spinal column
Ovary
Fallopian tube
varium

Ureter
Bladder

Symphysis pubis

Fig. 3. — *Posterior movement of ovary :* paramedian sagittal section. Pelvis of 2 1/2 month fetus (× 15).

In the urogenital sinus, two regions can be distinguished on either side of the openings of the Wolffian and Müllerian ducts.

— The cranial, or **urinary region,** was studied with the urinary system.

— The caudal, or **genital region,** will be examined here. This region may be considered in two parts:

— The interior, vertical portion is the *pelvic portion* of the urogenital sinus. In the female fetus, its cranial end contains ventrally the urethral orifice, and dorsally, the termination of the vaginal epithelial plate.

— The superficial, horizontal portion is the *phallic portion* of the urogenital sinus. It is bordered cranially by the genital tubercle, caudally by the urogenital membrane. After resorption of this membrane in the 9th week, the phallic portion of the urogenital sinus is open to the exterior (fig. 1 and 2).

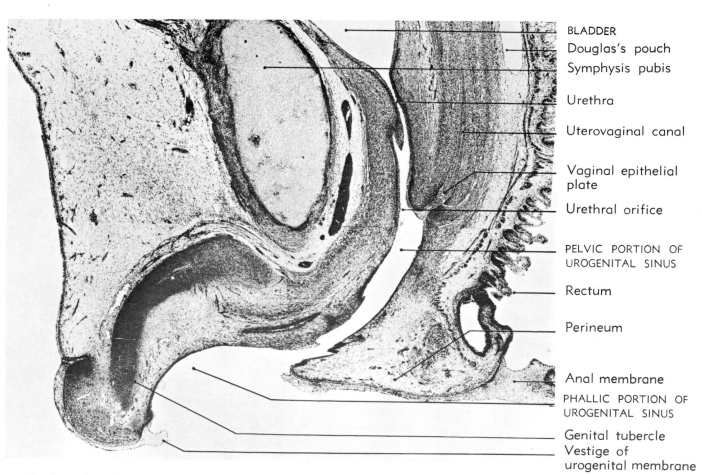

BLADDER
Douglas's pouch
Symphysis pubis

Urethra

Uterovaginal canal

Vaginal epithelial plate

Urethral orifice

PELVIC PORTION OF UROGENITAL SINUS

Rectum

Perineum

Anal membrane

PHALLIC PORTION OF UROGENITAL SINUS

Genital tubercle
Vestige of urogenital membrane

Fig. 1. — *Genital portion of female urogenital sinus after resorption of urogenital membrane.*
Median sagittal section. Fetus in 9th week ($\times$ 35).

OF GENITAL TRACT

Differentiation of the genital portion of the urogenital sinus in the female follows that of the urogenital excretory system. It begins in the 3rd month and parallels formation of the vagina and the external genital organs.

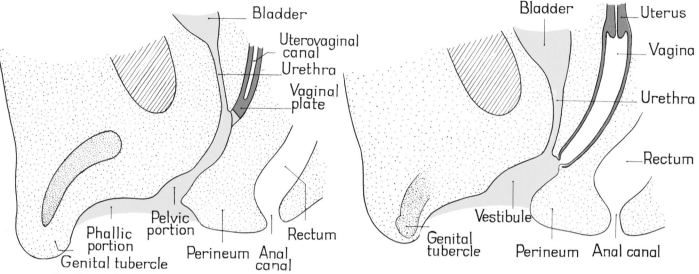

Fig. 2. — *Opening of urogenital membrane.*

Fig. 3. — *The definitive vestibule.*

The pelvic portion of the urogenital sinus becomes less and less deep, bringing to the surface the urethral orifice, or urinary meatus, and the hymen.

Finally, the pelvic portion is incorporated in the phallic portion, forming with it *the vestibule,* which is surrounded by the external genital organs (fig. 3 and 4).

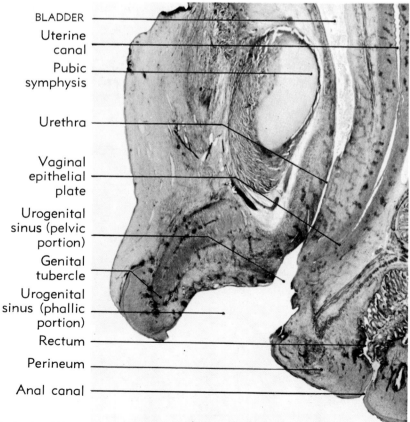

Fig. 4. — *Formation of vestibule* (× 11).

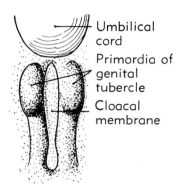

Fig. 1 *a*.

During the 3rd week (fig. 1 *a*), the cloacal membrane is very extended and its anterior end is level with the base of the umbilical cord. At this stage, the cloacal membrane is bordered laterally by two mesenchymal projections covered with ectoderm; these are the paired primordia of the genital tubercle.

At 4 weeks (fig. 1 *b*), the anterior end of the cloacal membrane retracts from the base of the umbilical cord. This permits formation of the anterior body wall caudal to the umbilicus. The paired primordia of the genital tubercle come together on the median line forming the genital tubercle. The cloacal fold, surrounding the cloacal membrane, further prolongs the genital tubercle.

At the same time, new formations appear: the genital swellings. These structures surround the genital tubercle and the cloacal fold.

At 7 weeks (fig. 1 *c*), the cloacal membrane is divided into the urogenital membrane anteriorly, and the anal membrane posteriorly, separated by the perineum. The cloacal fold is divided into the genital fold surrounding the urogenital membrane, and the anal fold circumscribing the ectodermal depression of the proctodeum.

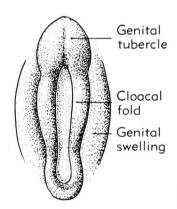

Fig. 1 *b*.

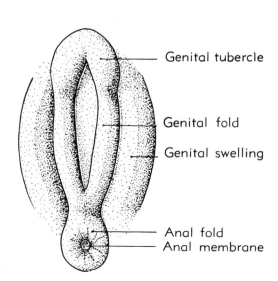

Fig. 1 *c*.

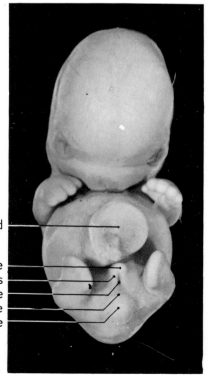

Fig. 2. — *Indifferent external genital organs.* Fetus, 2 months (× 5).

GENITAL ORGANS

In the 9th week (fig. 3), the urogenital membrane disappears, opening the phallic segment of the urogenital sinus to the exterior.

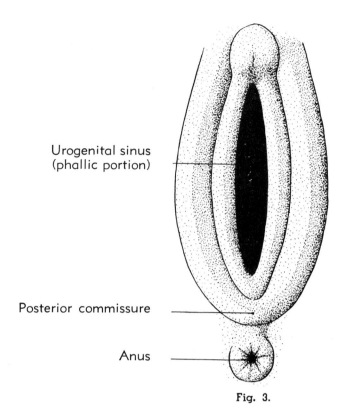

Urogenital sinus (phallic portion)

Posterior commissure

Anus

Fig. 3.

Differentiation of the external female genital organs takes place during the 3rd month and follows closely the primitive structures:

— The genital tubercle elongates only moderately and forms the *clitoris*. Erectile structures develop here.

— The urogenital sinus remains open to the exterior. Towards the interior of the vestibule, the urethra opens anteriorly, and the vagina posteriorly.

— Laterally, the vestibule is bordered by the genital folds which become *labia minora*.

— The genital swellings form the *labia majora*.

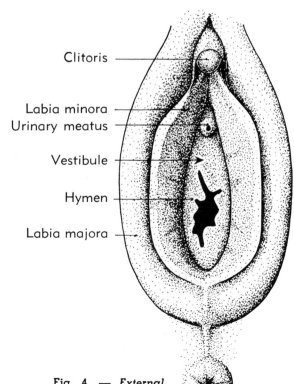

Clitoris

Labia minora
Urinary meatus

Vestibule

Hymen

Labia majora

Fig. 4. — *External female genital organs.*

GENETIC AND HORMONAL FACTORS

Until the 7th week, the gonad is undifferentiated. The sex of the embryo can be recognized only through its chromosomes: XX in the female embryo. At this time, however, the male or female chromosome constitution determines *differentiation of the genital gland* into a testis or an ovary.

Male differentiation of the genital receptors takes place successively for the urogenital excretory system, the urogenital sinus and the external genital organs. It is stimulated by testicular androgens. The external genital organs differentiate last, during the 3rd month.

Female differentiation of the genital receptors is related to absence of androgens. It follows quite closely the initial indifferent structures.

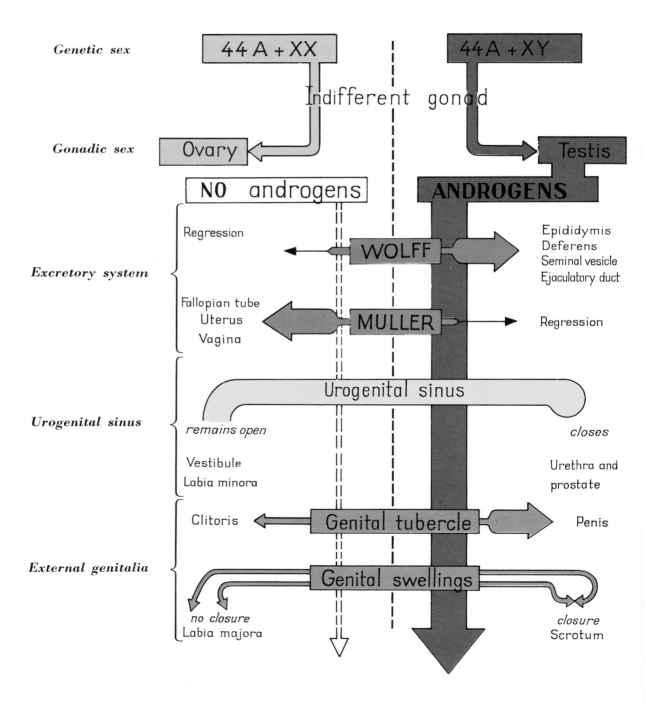

DIFFERENTIATION

SEXUAL ANOMALIES OF GENETIC ORIGIN

Alterations of the sex chromosomes may be transmitted by one of the parents (*gonadal dysgenesis*) or may occur in the embryo itself, even though the egg initially had a normal chromosome stock (*true hermaphroditism*).

Gonadal dysgenesis due to failure of disjunction of sex chromosomes during gametogenesis in one of the parents, may result in:

— *testicular dysgenesis of Klinefelter*, with male morphology and karyotype XXY;

— *ovarian agenesis of Turner*, with female morphology; here the karyotype has only a single sex chromosome, X, and is thus called XO.

The **true hermaphroditisms** are secondary to failure of disjunction of sex chromosomes during the first cleavage mitoses of the egg. These anomalies lead to the sex mosaics XY/XX or XY/XO. The relative quantitative importance of the male component (Y) in the mixed gland thus formed explains ultimate variations in androgenic effects, including different degrees of differentiation of the external genital organs, and subtle differences in somatic morphology.

SEXUAL ANOMALIES OF HORMONAL ORIGIN

Sexual anomalies of hormonal origin are seen in subjects with normal genetic constitution. The ambiguity of primary and secondary sexual characteristics leading to pseudohermaphroditism is related to somatic effects of abnormal androgen secretion (excess or deficiency).

Male pseudohermaphroditism is due to insufficient androgen secretion of an otherwise normal testis with a male XY karyotype.

A slight deficiency affects only the last stages of differentiation of the external genital organs: small penis, hypospadias, vulviform appearance of scrotum. General morphology, however, is masculine.

On the other hand, a severe deficiency allows persistence of the Müllerian system: a vagina and a uterus thus coexist with 2 normal deferent ducts. The testes are ectopic. The external genital organs, as well as general morphology, are of the female type.

Female pseudohermaphroditism is due to abnormal virilization of a female fetus with normal ovaries and an XX karyotype. The virilization may be of endogenous origin, by excessive androgenic secretion of the fetal adrenal, or of exogenous origin, related to maternal administration of synthetic progesterones or anabolic hormonal medications containing androgens.

The Müllerian system develops normally, but the androgens cause persistence of the Wolffian system and differentiation of the external genitalia toward the male: peniform clitoris, tendency toward closure of urogenital sinus, and coalescence of labia majora.

UTEROVAGINAL MALFORMATIONS

1. By partial or total failure of fusion of the terminal portion of the Müllerian ducts.

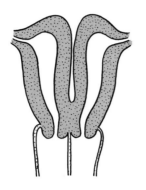 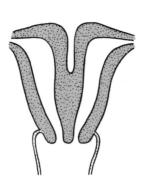 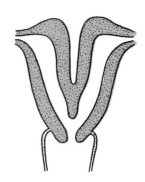

Fig. 1 *a*. — *Uterus didelphys with double vagina.* Fig. 1 *b*. — *Bicervical uterus bicornis.* Fig. 1 *c*. — *Unicervical uterus bicornis.*

2. By partial or total atresia of the terminal portion of one of both Müllerian ducts.

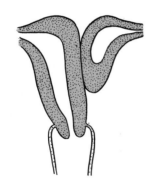 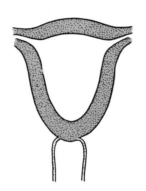 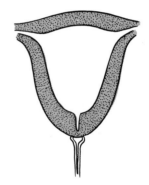

Fig. 1 *d*. — *Unilateral atresia: uterus bicornis unicollis: (rudimentary horn).* Fig. 1 *e*. *Partial bilateral atresia: atresia of cervix.* Fig. 1 *f*. *Partial bilateral atresia: atresia of vagina.*

3. By failure of resorption of uterovaginal septum after fusion of the Müllerian ducts.

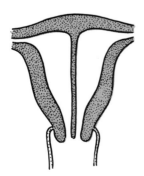 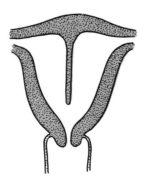 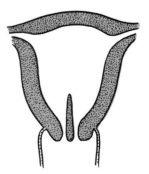

Fig. 1 *g*. — *Completely bilocular uterus.* Fig. 1 *h*. — *Bilocular unicervical uterus.* Fig. 1 *i*. — *Bilocular bicervical uterus.*

Fig. 1 *a-i*. — *Examples of uterovaginal malformations.* In the majority of cases, these malformations are completely latent, and are revealed only by chance through complications of pregnancy, or by hysterography. Only severe atresias are discerned earlier; these cause difficult therapeutic problems.

GENITAL SYSTEM

MIXED UROGENITAL MALFORMATIONS

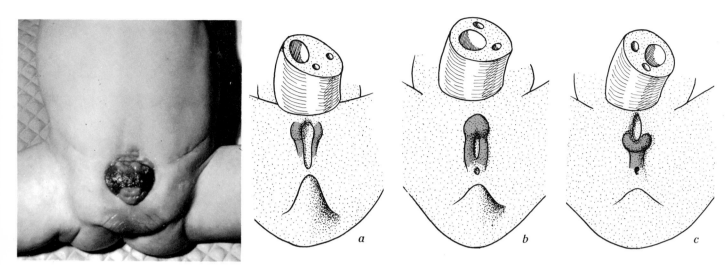

Fig. 2. — *Ectopia or exstrophy of the bladder.*

Fig. 3 a, b, c. — *Normal and abnormal development of the cloacal membrane.*

An abnormality of formation of the ventral body wall caudal to the umbilicus brings about a relatively frequent bladder anomaly which is difficult to treat : *exstrophy of the bladder.* In this case, the cloacal membrane does not retract normally towards the perineum, and the genital tubercles complete their more or less altered coalescence between its urogenital and its anal portions. Disappearance of the membrane in the 9th week thus exposes the posterior side of the bladder to the exterior, continuous with the rest of the lateral abdominal wall. Failure of formation of the urogenital groove, which depends on the same process, explains the frequent (but not obligatory) association of *epispadia,* opening of the urethra on the superior side of the penis or clitoris.

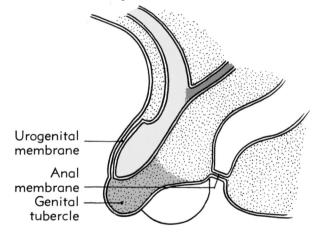

Urogenital membrane

Anal membrane

Genital tubercle

Fig. 4. — *Sagittal section showing formation of exstrophy of bladder and severe penile epispadia.*

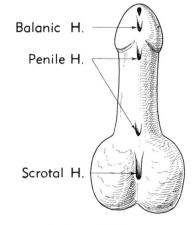

Balanic H.

Penile H.

Scrotal H.

Fig. 5. — *Different types of partial hypospadias.*

The urogenital groove, normally formed on the inferior side of the penis from a normally structured urogenital sinus, can still close abnormally, creating *hypospadia.*

All degrees can be seen, from balanic hypospadia (simple ectopia of the urethral meatus), to severe types where the urethra opens at the base of the penis or even in the perineal region. In these severe forms, there is always an anomaly associated with coalescence of the scrotal swellings giving the classic appearance of the vulviform hypospadias.

The blood and the cardiovascular system are derived from the mesoderm. They develop at the same time, beginning about the middle of the 3rd week.

It should be noted that the first blood and vascular elements appear at the *exterior of the embryo*, in the mesenchyme lining the yolk sac. However, this extraembryonic network rapidly blends with the intraembryonic circulation which appears a little later (beginning of the 4th week).

The yolk sac regresses at the end of the 2nd month, and with it its blood-forming islands. The hematopoietic function is then taken up by the liver.

PRIMITIVE BLOOD ISLANDS

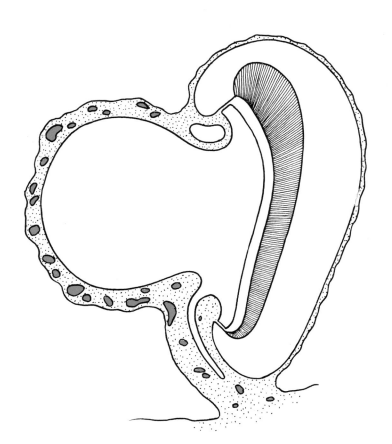

Fig. 1. — *Diagram of a human embryo of 3 weeks.* Appearance of islands of Wolff and Pander (in red) in the mesenchyme lining the yolk sac and allantois.

Towards the 18th-19th day, *clusters of mesenchymal cells* differentiate in the chorion, the connecting stalk, and the yolk sac wall. These clusters give rise to blood- and vascular-forming structures : the **islands of Wolff and Pander.**

Cells on the periphery of an island flatten and form *endothelial cells* which outline the vessels.

The central cells become free and give rise to the blood cells. These parent cells or *hemocytoblasts* are the origin of three lines of blood cells, but at this stage, they give rise essentially to nucleated red cells (megaloblasts).

SYSTEM

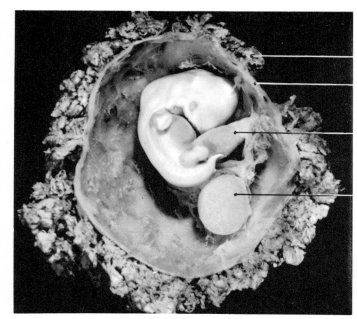

Placenta

Chorion

Umbilical cord

YOLK SAC

Fig. 2. — *Fetal membranes: placenta and yolk sac.* Human embryo of 34 days in opened embryonic vesicle (× 6).

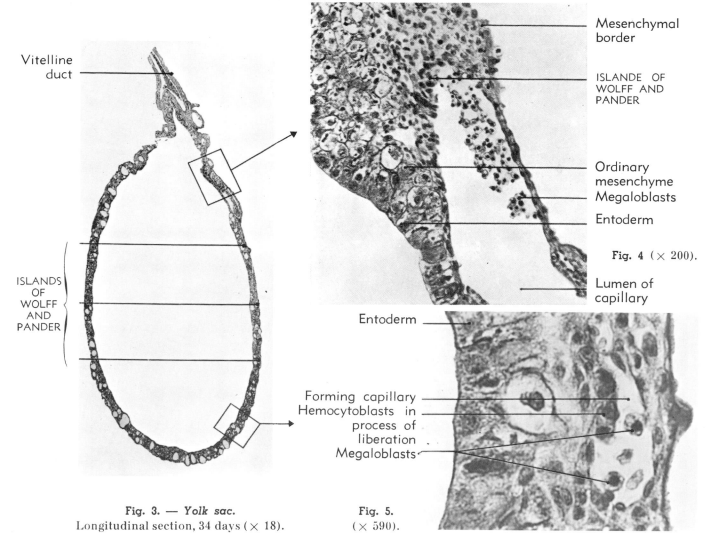

Vitelline duct

ISLANDS OF WOLFF AND PANDER

Fig. 3. — *Yolk sac.*
Longitudinal section, 34 days (× 18).

Mesenchymal border

ISLANDE OF WOLFF AND PANDER

Ordinary mesenchyme

Megaloblasts

Entoderm

Fig. 4 (× 200).

Lumen of capillary

Entoderm

Forming capillary
Hemocytoblasts in process of liberation
Megaloblasts

Fig. 5.
(× 590).

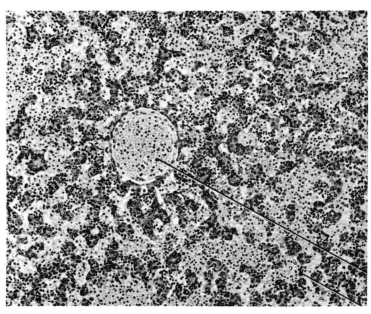

The yolk sac capillaries form a network drained by the *vitelline veins.*

These veins flow directly into the venous sinus of the heart, forming first an anastomotic network around the duodenum, then crossing the *septum transversum* (see pp. 130 and 131).

In the middle of the 3rd week (at the same time that vascular primordia appear generally) the hepatic primordium, of entodermal origin, begins to invade the septum transversum.

Centrolobular vein

Sinusoidal and erythroblastic capillaries

Fig. 1. — *Hematopoietic liver.*
Human liver. Fetus of 2 months (× 80).

By proliferation, the hepatic epithelial cords surround the vitelline veins, and fragment them into a multitude of *sinusoidal capillaries.*

Extension of proliferation to the entire septum transversum carries the same process to the umbilical veins.

Next, the hepatic cells, hepatocytes, become arranged into cords surrounding the sinusoidal capillaries (fig. 2).

Hepatic hematopoiesis begins during the 2nd month and reaches its maximum in the 3rd month, then decreases and ceases about the 7th month. Hematopoiesis is assumed by the bone marrow, which becomes functional beginning with the 4th month (fig. 4).

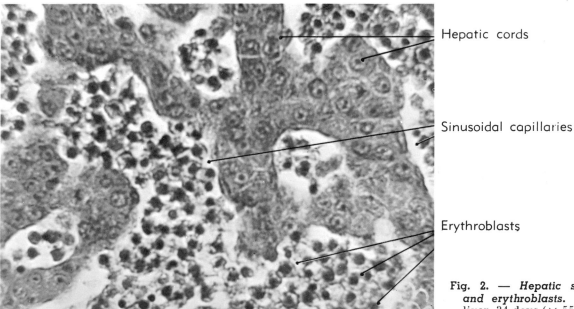

Hepatic cords

Sinusoidal capillaries

Erythroblasts

Fig. 2. — *Hepatic sinusoids and erythroblasts.* Human liver, 34 days (× 550).

POIESIS

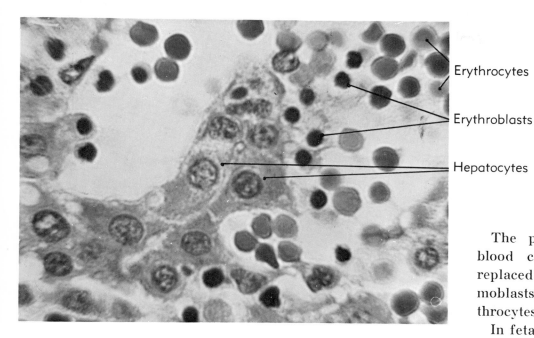

Fig. 3. — *Erythrocytes and erythroblasts.*
Human liver.   Embryo of 45 days (× 1,200).

The primitive nucleated red blood cells (megaloblasts) are replaced by erythroblasts (normoblasts), then by mature erythrocytes without nuclei.

In fetal-maternal blood incompatibility, where there is immunization of the mother against the red blood cells of her fetus, the maternal antibodies destroy the fetal red blood cells. The fetal organism reacts against the increasing anemia by intense erythropoiesis. The liver retains its hematopoietic role beyond the 7th month and puts red blood cells into circulation even before their complete maturation. The presence of erythroblasts in the blood at birth is one of the characteristic signs of hemolytic disease (see Volume I).

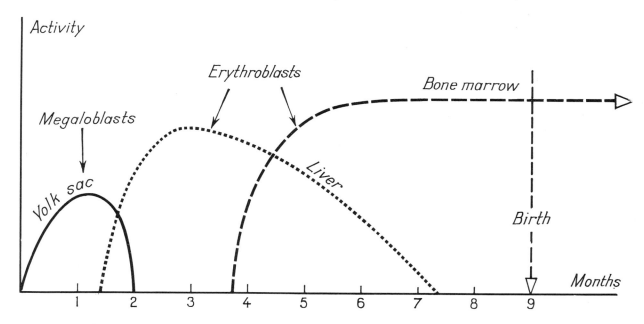

Fig. 4. — *Chronology of normal hematopoiesis.*
Note the importance of the bone marrow after the 4th month.

The circulatory system undergoes many important rearrangements during its development.

These complex modifications of the vascular plan are related to function: in the embryo, as in the adult, the organs necessary for survival, having a great deal of metabolic activity, have priority. These are the organs of nutrition and of excretion.

The transition from fetal to autonomous life, marked by physiological changes, also leads to profound circulatory modifications.

Three essential stages may be distinguished:

— the *vitelline stage*, where the embryo lives on its reserves (which are small);

— the *placental stage*, where an intermediary organ (the placenta) develops between the maternal and fetal organisms;

— the *neonatal stage*, where the organism assumes its survival autonomously.

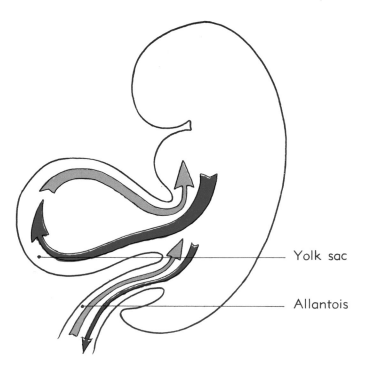

Yolk sac

Allantois

Fig. 1. — *Vitelline stage.* Circulatory network of an embryo of about 4 weeks.

Vitelline stage (fig. 1)
(from the 3rd week to the beginning of the 2nd month).

— Vitelline circulation (yolk sac) is predominant.

— Primitive intraembryonic circulation and allantoic circulation are forming.

CIRCULATORY SYSTEM

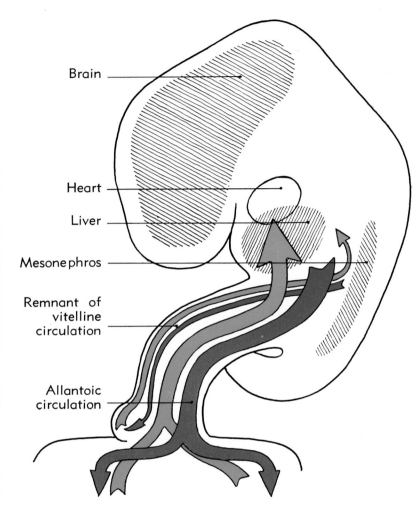

Brain

Heart

Liver

Mesonephros

Remnant of
vitelline
circulation

Allantoic
circulation

Fig. 2. — *Placental stage.*

Placental stage (fig. 2)
(from the end of the 1st month to birth).

— The vitelline circulation disappears at the end of the 2nd month. From its only vestige arise the superior mesenteric vessels.

— Allantoic circulation becomes *placental* and is predominant after the 30th day.

It is accomplished by the *umbilical vessels,* and is responsible for oxygenation, nutrition, and filtration.

— Intraembryonic circulation is marked by special enlargement of the liver, the brain, and the mesonephros.

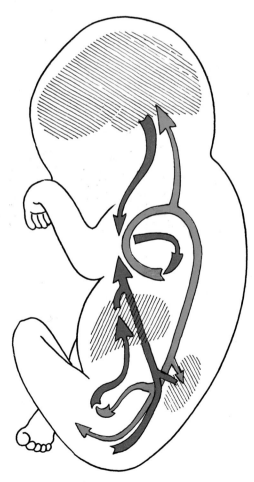

Neonatal stage
(fig. 3).

Placental circulation is interrupted.

Its role is taken over in neonatal circulation by specialized organs:

— a special pulmonary area, well developed anatomically, begins to function for oxygenation;

— the metanephros, functional since the 3rd month, is responsible for filtration;

— the mesenteric network which drains the digestive tract insures nutrition.

Fig. 3. — *Neonatal stage.*

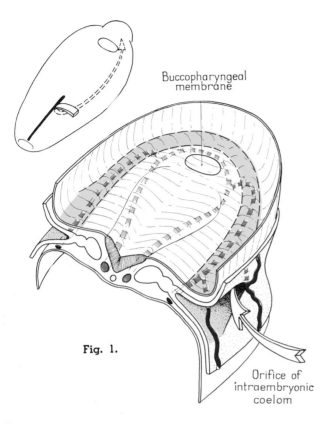

Buccopharyngeal membrane

Fig. 1.

Orifice of intraembryonic coelom

During gastrulation (see Volume I), part of the mesoderm migrates from the primitive streak to the pharyngeal membrane. It unites with its pair from the opposite side to form the cardiac primordium.

Cleavage of the lateral plate by the coelom reaches this region, bringing about differentiation of the splanchnopleure and the somatopleure. These form the walls of the future pericardial cavity.

After the 20th day, islands appear in the splanchnopleure, then by confluence, two tubes called **endocardial tubes** are formed (fig. 1 and 2).

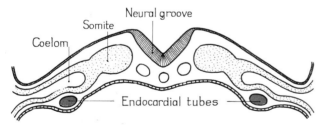

Neural groove

Somite

Coelom

Endocardial tubes

Fig. 2. — *Endocardial tubes in the splanchnopleure.*

While the embryo is undergoing cephalocaudal flexion (see Volume I), these two tubes approach each other on the midline. Closure of the foregut places them in a ventral position (fig. 3).

About the 22nd day, the two endocardial tubes come together, then fuse in the craniocaudal direction (fig. 4 and 5). This fusion is succeeded by disappearance of the ventral mesocardium. Partial disappearance of the dorsal mesocardium then follows.

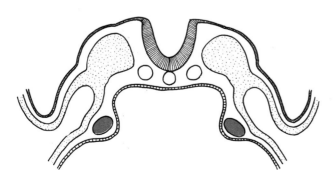

Fig. 3. — *Embryonic cephalocaudal flexion.*

OF THE HEART

TUBE

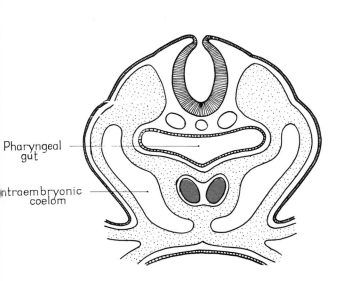

Pharyngeal gut

ntraembryonic coelom

Fig. 4. — *Joining of tubes.*

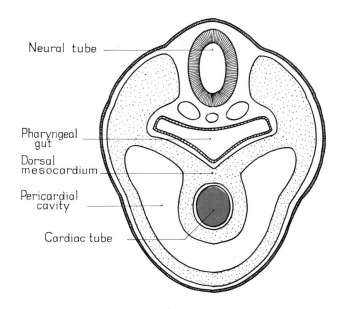

Neural tube

Pharyngeal gut

Dorsal mesocardium

Pericardial cavity

Cardiac tube

Fig. 5. — *Fusion into a median tube.*

The single median cardiac tube begins to beat about the 23rd day. It grows considerably in the pericardial cavity which does not undergo the same increase in size: it must therefore undergo a complex folding.

Between the 27th and 29th days, true embryonic circulation is established.

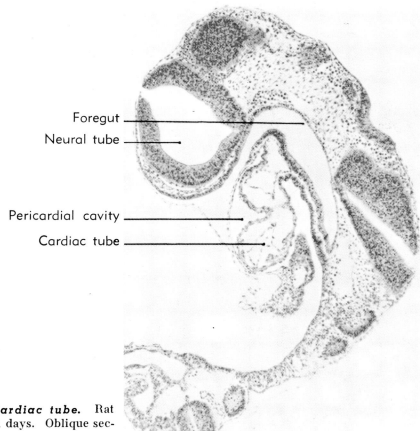

Foregut

Neural tube

Pericardial cavity

Cardiac tube

Fig. 6. — *Cardiac tube.* Rat embryo, 11 days. Oblique section (× 80).

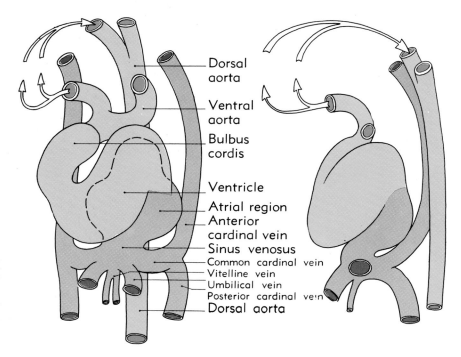

Dorsal aorta

Ventral aorta

Bulbus cordis

Ventricle

Atrial region

Anterior cardinal vein

Sinus venosus

Common cardinal vein

Vitelline vein

Umbilical vein

Posterior cardinal vein

Dorsal aorta

Fig. 1. — Cardiac tube at 25th day.

II. — AURICULOVENTRICULAR

By the 25th day, the cardiac tube is folded in the pericardial cavity. It is comprised of:

— the sinus venosus, into whose horns enter the vitelline veins, the umbilical veins, and the common cardinal veins;

— the atrial region, which communicates with the ventricle by the atrioventricular canal;

— the ventricular region;

— the bulbus cordis, which is a prolongation of the ventricle, and gives rise to the aortic roots.

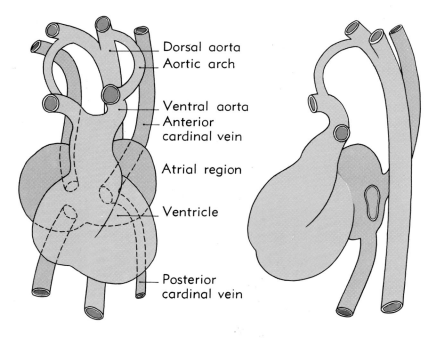

Dorsal aorta

Aortic arch

Ventral aorta

Anterior cardinal vein

Atrial region

Ventricle

Posterior cardinal vein

Fig. 2. — Cardiac tube at 28th day.

By the 28th day, the atrial region has become a large cavity dorsal to the ventricular region, and divided into 2 pouches, the right and left atria.

At this time, the ventricle is bounded by the bulbus cordis ventrally and the atria dorsally. The fold between the bulbus cordis and ventricle rapidly disappears.

SEPTATION

The separation between atria and ventricle increases, shrinking the atrioventricular canal. On the ventral and dorsal walls of the canal there now appear thickenings, the 2 endocardial cushions, which move toward each other and finally fuse, between the **35th and the 40th day,** to form the primitive interventricular septum.

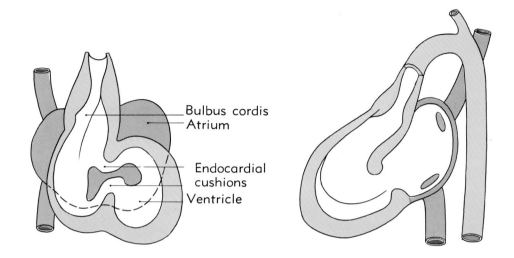

Fig. 3. — *Cardiac tube at 35th day.*

By the **40th day,** the atrioventricular canal is divided into two auriculoventricular orifices, right and left.

The mesenchyme surrounding each orifice proliferates and forms the atrioventricular valves:

— the mitral valve at left;

— the tricuspid valve at right.

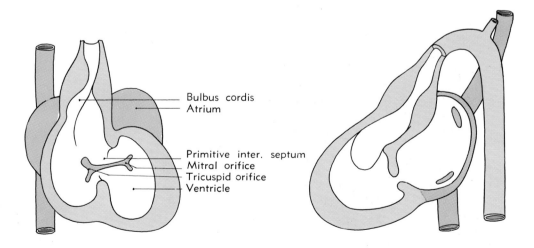

Fig. 4. — *Cardiac tube at 40th day.*

Auricular septation begins during the 5th week.

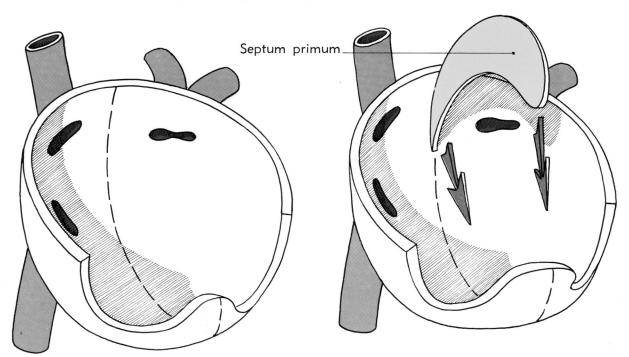

Septum primum

Fig. 1. — *The single atrium: first stage.* In order to provide better orientation, the diagram shows the venous system fully formed. In reality, at this stage only the common cardinal veins and the vitelline and umbilical veins can be seen.

Fig. 2. — *Appearance on the posterosuperior wall of a thin sickle-shaped septum.* Its points converge toward the septum intermedium. *This is the septum primum.*

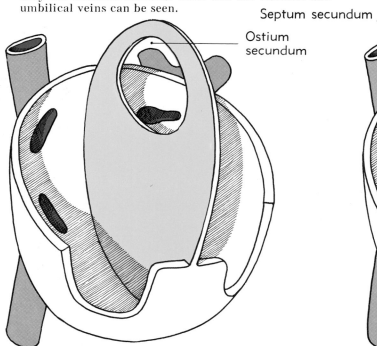

Septum secundum

Ostium secundum

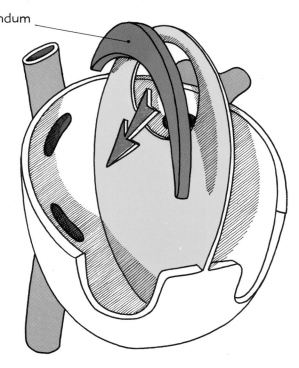

Fig. 5. — When the ostium primum is closed, the *ostium secundum* maintains free passage between the two atria.

Fig. 6. — *To the right of the delicate septum primum,* on the anterosuperior wall, a thick septum appears. Its points converge toward the opening of the inferior vena cava. This is the *septum secundum* (appearing in the 7th week).

This series of diagrams shows the atrial region cut horizontally with its upper portion removed. The openings shown in the anterior wall represent the atrioventricular orifices, separated by the primitive interauricular septum.

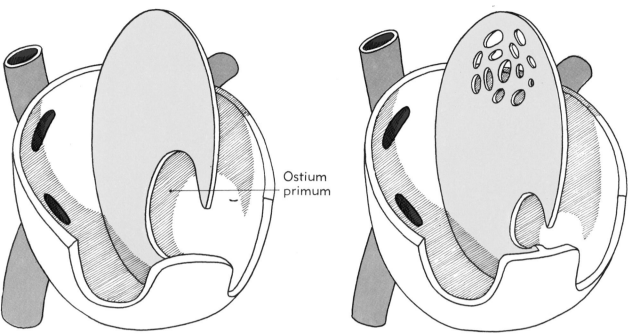

Fig. 3. — *The septum primum delimits, with the primitive interauricular septum, a temporary orifice, the ostium primum,* which rapidly gets smaller.

Fig. 4. — During closure of the ostium primum, *small openings appear in the upper portion of the septum primum.* These orifices merge to form the *ostium secundum.*

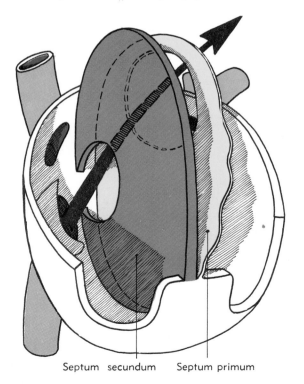

Fig. 7. — *The septum secundum covers the ostium secundum but remains incomplete.* There is an oval-shaped passage in the interauricular septum directly in the path of the blood coming from the inferior vena cava (black arrow). This is the *foramen ovale.*

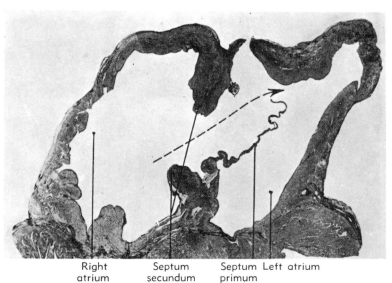

Fig. 8. — *Very oblique section of the interauricular septum through the foramen ovale.* Fetus, 5 months.

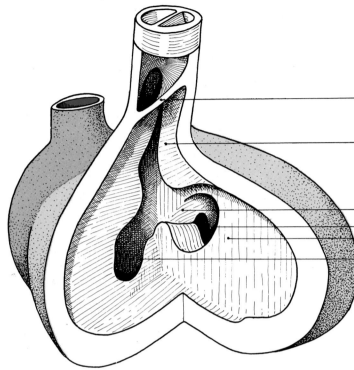

Fig. 1. — *Interventricular septum.*

— Aorticopulmonary septum

— Bulbus cordis

— Primitive interventricular septum
— Mitral orifice
— Incomplete interventricular septum
— Tricuspid orifice

In the 5th week (at the same time that the interauricular septum is forming), a crest appears on the anterior ventricular wall, almost in its median plane. This is the primordium of the interventricular septum (fig. 1).

The interventricular septum is incomplete; interventricular communication persists in the bulbus.

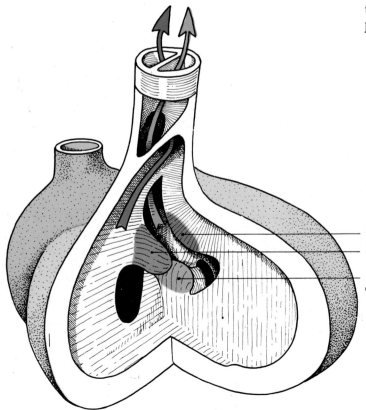

Fig. 2. — *The aorticopulmonary septum.*

Left truncoconal ridge
Right truncoconal ridge

Proliferation of posterior atrioventricular endocardial cushion.

During the 5th week, the 6th aortic arch appears and contributes to formation of the pulmonary arteries. Just cephalic to the 6th arch, the bulbus cordis thickens into 2 ridges: the truncoconal ridges (fig. 2).

SEPTATION

As the truncoconal ridges grow, they descend in a spiral on the walls of the bulbus in the direction of the ventricles. They soon fuse, forming the aorticopulmonary septum, which separates definitively the aorta and the pulmonary artery. As a result of the spiral form of the septum, the aorta and pulmonary artery twist around each other.

Septation is completed by closure of the interventricular communication by :

— a proliferation of the right truncoconal ridge near the tricuspid orifice;

— a proliferation of the left truncoconal ridge near the mitral orifice;

— a proliferation of the posterior endocardial cushion.

Fusion of these three outgrowths forms the membranous part of the interventricular septum (fig. 2 and 3), and is completed toward the end of the 2nd month.

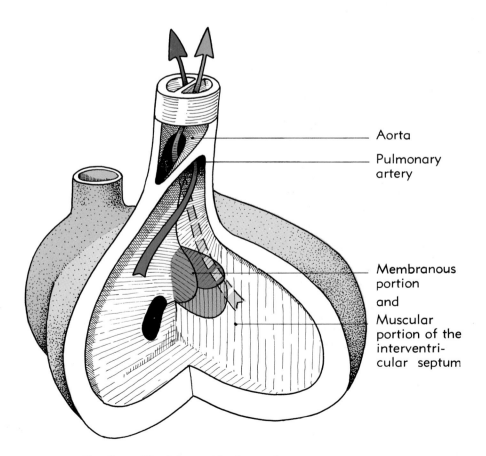

Aorta

Pulmonary artery

Membranous portion
and
Muscular portion of the interventricular septum

Fig. 3. — *The interventricular septum.*

(These dates are not absolute;
they are only statistical means.)

Week	Days	Somites	Length in mm
3	15		
	16		
	17		
	18		
	19		
	20	1	1,5
	21	4	
4	22	7	
	23	10	
	24	13	2
	25	15	
	26	20	3
	27		
	28	25	4
5	29		
	30	28	
	31		
	32		5
	33		
	34		6,5
	35		
6	36		8
	37		
	38		
	39		
	40		
	41		
	42		13
7	43		
	44		
	45		
	46		
	47		
	48		
	49		20

Cardiogenic plate.
Endocardial tubes.
Fusing endocardial tubes.
Single median tube.

Cardiac loop.
Single atrium.

First contractions (ineffective)

Bilobed atrium.

Beginnings of circulation

Septum primum.

Septum intermedium.

Auriculoventricular orifices (3-chambered heart).

Septum secundum.

Completed septum inferius.
Septation of bulbus and ventricle.

Divided truncus arteriosus.

Four-chambered heart.
Absorption of pulmonary veins.

OF CARDIAC DEVELOPMENT

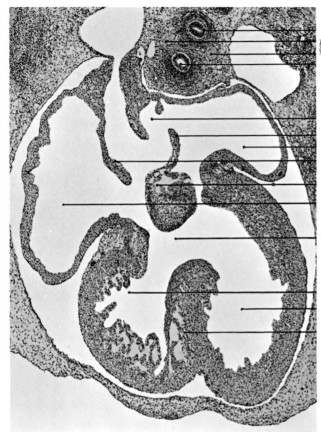

Esophagus
Vagus nerves
Trachea

Ostium secundum
Septum primum
Left atrium
Venous valve

Septum intermedium

Right atrium

Interventricular communication
(later closed by the membranous septum)

Right ventricle
Left ventricle
Septum inferius

Fig. 1. — *Horizontal section showing the 4 cardiac chambers.* Human embryo, 34 days (× 43).

Right atrium

Venous valves

Septum secundum
Foramen ovale
Septum primum
Tricuspid valve

Right ventricle

Interventricular septum
Left atrium
Mitral valve

Left auricle

Left ventricle

Fig. 2. — *Longitudinal section.* Heart of rat fetus at term (× 20).

The initial circulatory system is achieved by the almost simultaneous formation of the heart and three networks: *intraembryonic, vitelline,* and *umbilicoallantoic.*

These vascular networks form from vascular blood islands arising in the mesenchyme. The islands hollow, then combine to form a capillary plexus in which certain branches predominate from an early stage. Only these persist. Later these primitive vessels derive their muscle and connective tissue layers from the neighboring mesenchyme.

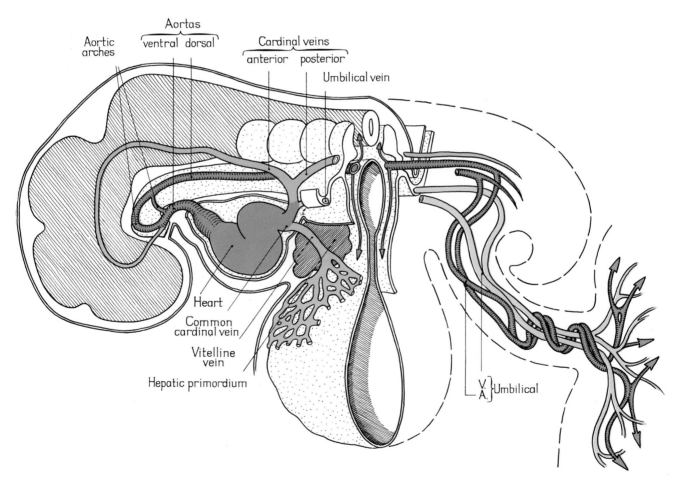

Fig. 1. — *Overall view of primitive vascular system.*
Human embryo, 25 days.

CIRCULATORY NETWORKS

*1. **The intraembryonic vascular network.*** — *a*) **Arteries.** — The ventral arteries, the first aortic arches, and the dorsal aortas are continuous. In the anterior region, in each branchial arch, 5 pairs of aortic arches form *successively,* joining the ventral to the dorsal aortas. The anterior arches disappear as the posterior ones develop.

The dorsal aortas extend from the cranial to the caudal region, and put forth *paired segmental arteries* corresponding to the somites.

The segmental arteries consist of a dorsal series vascularizing the neural tube, and a ventral series surrounding the primitive gut.

Some ventral arteries make a junction with the extraembryonic vascular network:

— the *omphalomesenteric arteries* continue as *vitelline arteries* in the vascular system of the yolk sac;

— the *allantoic or umbilical arteries* feed the placental network.

b) **Veins.** — The paired anterior and posterior *cardinal veins* also develop in the same way, but slightly later than the aortas.

In the heart, they join to give the common cardinal veins, which open in the sinus venosus, close to the vitelline and umbilical veins.

*2. **The vitelline vascular network*** develops on the yolk sac surface, especially in its caudal half, and reforms into four large vessels:

— *the vitelline arteries,* whose proximal portion is the omphalomesenteric arteries;

— *the vitelline veins,* which flow ventrally in the embryo into the sinus venosus.

*3. **The placental vascular network,*** developed in the mesenchyme around the allantois is also resolved into four large vessels:

— *the two allantoic or umbilical arteries,* which are actually two of the posterior segmental arteries of the aorta;

— *two umbilical veins,* which flow into the sinus venosus. These two veins come together in a single trunk at the level of the umbilical cord.

The arterial system thus formed undergoes several modifications. These are:

— minimal in the *posterior region;*

— basic in the *middle portion:* fusion of the 2 dorsal aortas into a single aorta;

— complex and tiered in the *anterior region:* the aortic arches.

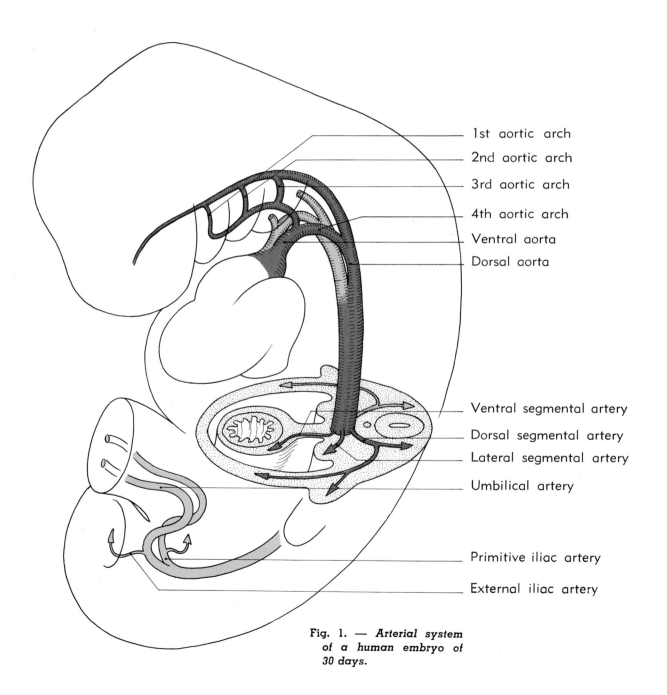

1st aortic arch
2nd aortic arch
3rd aortic arch
4th aortic arch
Ventral aorta
Dorsal aorta

Ventral segmental artery
Dorsal segmental artery
Lateral segmental artery
Umbilical artery

Primitive iliac artery
External iliac artery

Fig. 1. — *Arterial system of a human embryo of 30 days.*

ARTERIAL SYSTEM

I. — IN THE POSTERIOR REGION

The paired umbilical arteries arise from a dorsal aorta at the posterior extremity of the ventral segmental arteries.

These arteries remain paired. During growth of the embryo, their point of origin moves slightly in the caudal direction, and they put forth a small external branch to the lower limbs.

At birth, placental circulation is interrupted. The umbilical arteries become fibrous over most of their length. Their proximal portion gives rise to the primitive iliac, hypogastric, and superior vesical arteries. The branch destined for the lower limb becomes the external iliac artery.

II. — IN THE MIDDLE REGION

About the 4th week, the 2 dorsal aortas approach and fuse, first in the middle portion, then cranially up to the 8th segmental artery, and caudally to the posterior end. The single dorsal aorta is then formed (middle of 5th week).

The paired **ventral segmental arteries** approach each other on the midline in the mesentery, and some fuse into a median vessel. In this way 3 visceral arterial systems appear:

— celiac trunk;

— superior mesenteric artery, which derives from a special segmental artery, the right omphalomesenteric artery after regression of its vitelline portion (the left disappears entirely);

— inferior mesenteric artery.

Temporary longitudinal anastomoses result in caudal movement of the origins of these arteries. The final level is reached at the end of the 2nd month.

The **dorsal segmental arteries,** in contrast, remain paired. At first they supply only the neural tube. Their somatic branches, however, grow considerably, and finally predominate. Some dorsal segmental arteries persist, for example, the inter-costal arteries.

The **lateral segmental arteries,** in 2 symmetrical series, provide a rich vascularization to the mesonephros and the gonad.

Theoretically, six pairs of aortic arches are formed. In fact, however, the 5th pair is only a temporary doubling of the 4th pair. *These arches form successively, and are never all present at the same time.*

The 1st aortic arch is formed by the curving of the ventral aorta into the primitive dorsal aorta. It is hidden in the mandibular arch. It participates in formation of the internal maxillary artery.

The 2nd aortic arch appears in the middle of the 4th week. It crosses the 2nd branchial arch and gives rise to the tympanic and the hyoid arteries.

These two arches regress rapidly; they are no longer visible after the 31st day.

The 3rd aortic arch appears at the end of the 4th week. From it is formed the proximal part of the internal carotid. The *internal carotids,* which are short *cephalic prolongations of the primitive dorsal aortas,* are associated with development of the brain (see Volume III). They are attached secondarily to a segment of the primitive ventral aorta which forms the *primitive carotid* artery.

The cephalic prolongation of the primitive ventral aorta will be the *external carotid.*

The 4th arch also appears at the end of the 4th week, shortly after the 3rd arch. Its fate is different on the right and left sides of the embryo.

— ON THE LEFT: it persists as the *aortic arch;* this grows considerably and is continuous with the primitive left dorsal aorta. The left subclavian, or 7th segmental artery, arises directly from the aorta.

— ON THE RIGHT: the 4th arch forms the proximal part of the right subclavian and is continuous with the 7th segmental artery. The caudal part of the right primitive dorsal aorta disappears.

The short portion of the right primitive ventral aorta, which persists between the 4th and 6th arches, forms the *brachiocephalic arterial trunk* and the *first part of the aortic arch.*

The 6th arch appears in the middle of the 5th week, and forms the right and left pulmonary arteries. When pulmonary vascularization is established, the communication with the corresponding primitive dorsal aorta regresses.

— ON THE RIGHT, regression is total.

— ON THE LEFT, the communication persists until birth. This is the *ductus arteriosus,* which diverts pulmonary blood into the aorta. First functional, then anatomical, closure of the ductus arteriosus takes place in the neonatal period.

THE AORTIC ARCHES

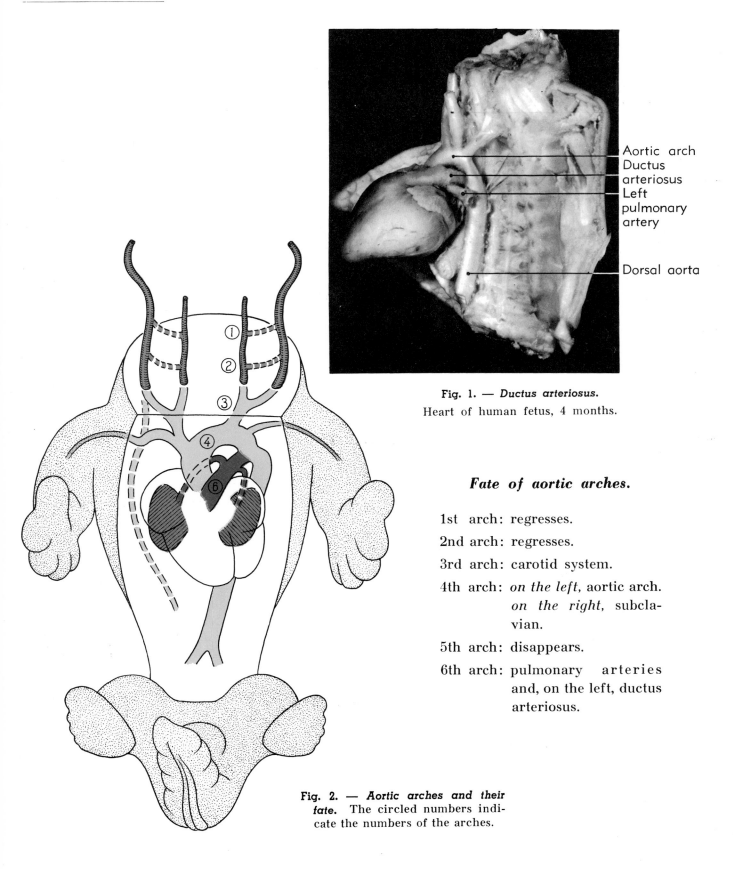

Fig. 1. — *Ductus arteriosus.*
Heart of human fetus, 4 months.

Aortic arch
Ductus arteriosus
Left pulmonary artery
Dorsal aorta

Fate of aortic arches.

1st arch: regresses.

2nd arch: regresses.

3rd arch: carotid system.

4th arch: *on the left,* aortic arch.
on the right, subclavian.

5th arch: disappears.

6th arch: pulmonary arteries and, on the left, ductus arteriosus.

Fig. 2. — *Aortic arches and their fate.* The circled numbers indicate the numbers of the arches.

I. — PRIMITIVE VENOUS NETWORKS

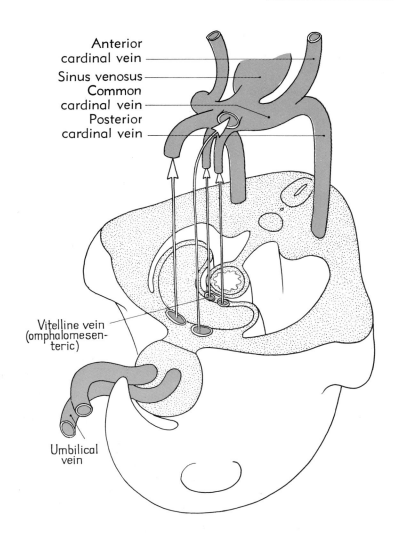

Anterior
cardinal vein
Sinus venosus
Common
cardinal vein
Posterior
cardinal vein

Vitelline vein
(omphalomesen-
teric)

Umbilical
vein

Fig. 1. — *The venous networks
in the 4th week.*

These networks are initially paired
and symmetrical, but by a system of
transverse anastomoses, they are con-
verted into single principal trunks in
the right half of the embryo.

In the 4th week, the venous system of the
embryo consists of (fig. 1):

a) **A dorsal systemic network,** carrying all
the *intraembryonic* blood, formed by the
anterior and posterior cardinal veins which
reach the venous sinus through the common cardinal veins.

b) **A double nutritional network** carrying
the extraembryonic blood:

— the omphalomesenteric system for
blood coming from the yolk sac;

— the umbilicoallantoic system for blood
coming from the placenta.

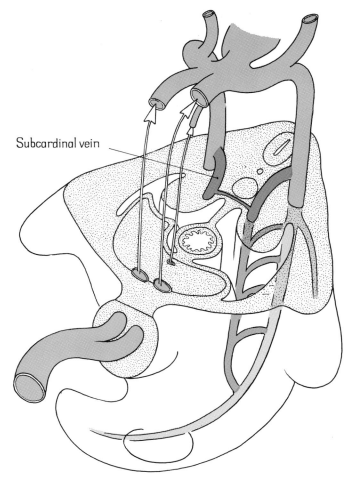

Subcardinal vein

Fig. 2. — *The venous networks in the 6th week.*

VENOUS SYSTEM

II. — DEVELOPMENT OF THE SUPERIOR VENA CAVA

The superior vena cava is formed later than the inferior vena cava, but its development is simpler.

— In the 8th week (fig. 3), a large anastomosis derived from the thymic and thyroid veins channels the blood from the left superior cardinal vein towards the right. This is the future *left brachiocephalic venous trunk.*

— Above this anastomosis, the anterior cardinal veins become the *internal jugulars.*

— the anterior veins of the mandibular region give rise to the *external jugular.*

— The venous plexes of the upper limb fuse to give the *subclavian vein.* This vein originally opens into the posterior cardinal vein, but as the heart shifts caudally, the subclavian finally transfers into the anterior cardinal vein.

The left anterior cardinal vein persists only as a short segment forming the *left superior intercostal vein.*

The left common cardinal vein persists only as a short segment forming the *coronary sinus venosus.*

The superior vena cava is finally formed by the right common cardinal vein and the proximal portion of the right anterior cardinal vein (see fig. 1 and 2, pp. 128 and 129).

Malformations of this simple system are rare. Nevertheless, the following have been described:

— left superior vena cava;

— double superior vena cava;

— abnormal pulmonary venous return, draining in the superior vena cava or the right atrium.

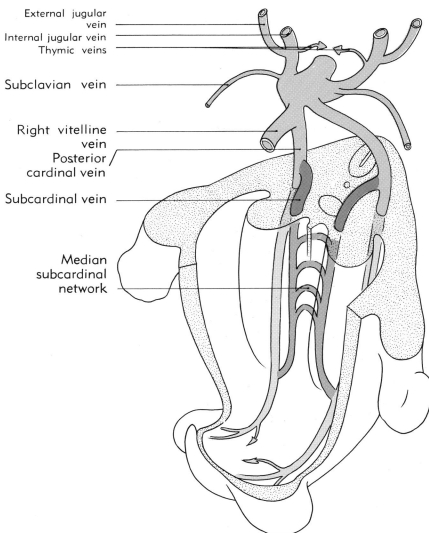

External jugular vein
Internal jugular vein
Thymic veins

Subclavian vein

Right vitelline vein
Posterior cardinal vein

Subcardinal vein

Median subcardinal network

Fig. 3. — *The venous networks in the 8th week.*

Several successive networks participate in the formation of the inferior vena cava. They predominate temporarily, then regress and remain only partially in the definitive system.

During the 4th week, the mesonephros grows considerably, and becomes highly vascularized. Although initially it is drained only by the posterior cardinal veins, after the 4th week a new system takes over, the **subcardinal network** formed by the internal veins of the Wolffian body (see fig. 2 and 3, pp. 126 and 127).

The internal veins of the Wolffian body are widely anastomosed:

— with the initial posterior cardinal network; and

— with each other, forming the median subcardinal network, which soon predominates. It takes over the posterior cardinal system which disappears in the middle region.

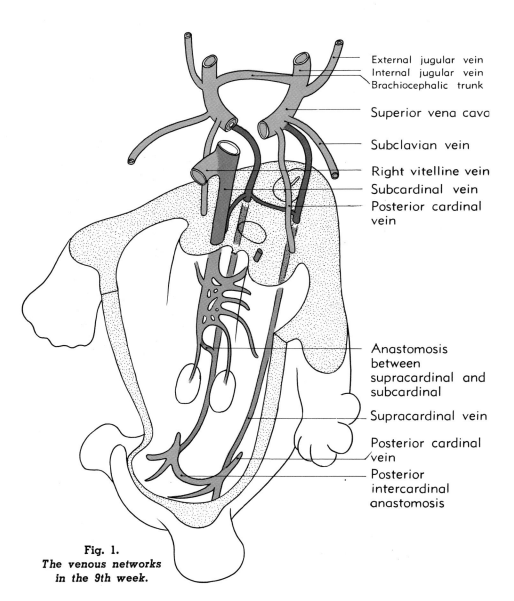

External jugular vein
Internal jugular vein
Brachiocephalic trunk

Superior vena cava

Subclavian vein

Right vitelline vein
Subcardinal vein
Posterior cardinal vein

Anastomosis between supracardinal and subcardinal

Supracardinal vein

Posterior cardinal vein

Posterior intercardinal anastomosis

Fig. 1.
The venous networks in the 9th week.

— *The subcardinal sinus* persists in the form of the left renal vein.

— The anterior segment of the *left subcardinal vein* disappears. Its posterior segment forms the left gonadal vein.

— *The right subcardinal vein* forms the right gonadal vein, and the pararenal segment of the definitive inferior vena cava. Cranially, it continues with the mesenteric segment and the hepatic segment derived from the hepatic vein (proximal right vitelline) and hepatic sinusoids.

INFERIOR VENA CAVA

During the 6th and the 7th weeks, a supplementary dorsal network is formed, the **supracardinal system,** which is parallel to the paravertebral sympathetic chain and opens into the proximal segment of the posterior cardinal veins.

Anastomoses are established:
— between the 2 supracardinal veins;
— between the supracardinals and the subcardinals (on the right);
— between the extremities of the posterior cardinal veins.

The left supracardinal vein becomes the hemiazygos vein and is drained towards the right by the transverse anastomosis which becomes interazygos.

The right supracardinal vein becomes the major azygos vein, which opens in the right anterior cardinal vein. Caudally, it drains the 2 iliac veins and thus becomes the prerenal portion of the definitive inferior vena cava (fig. 1, p. 128).

The definitive inferior vena cava is thus composed of the following parts (in caudocranial order):
— the posterior intercardinal anastomosis;
— the caudal segment of the right supracardinal;
— the right anastomosis between supracardinal and subcardinal;
— a segment of the right subcardinal;
— the anastomosis between the right subcardinal and right vitelline;
— the terminal portion of the right vitelline.

A system as complex as this permits formation of many *anomalies.* The most conspicuous of these is agenesis of the inferior vena cava. However, even in the most pronounced malformations, one of the constituent networks always substitutes. Thus, no clinical syndrome of caval malformation is recognized.

An abnormality of position can, in certain cases, affect neighboring organs, especially the ureter, which may be compressed and produce hydronephrosis.

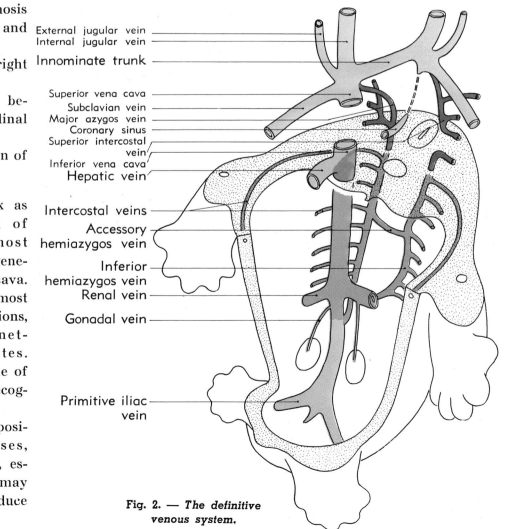

External jugular vein
Internal jugular vein
Innominate trunk
Superior vena cava
Subclavian vein
Major azygos vein
Coronary sinus
Superior intercostal vein
Inferior vena cava
Hepatic vein
Intercostal veins
Accessory hemiazygos vein
Inferior hemiazygos vein
Renal vein
Gonadal vein
Primitive iliac vein

Fig. 2. — *The definitive venous system.*

The vitelline veins (or omphalomesenterics) connected to the digestive tube constitute an anastomotic network around the duodenum, then cross the septum transversum (fig. 1).

Proliferation of the entodermal cords forming the hepatic primordium fragments the vitelline veins into a vascular labyrinth: the hepatic sinusoids. When the yolk sac disappears, the vitelline veins regress almost totally and persist only in their mesenteric branches.

Caudal to the liver, the anastomotic network of the vitelline veins fuses into a single trunk, the portal vein (fig. 2).

Cranial to the liver, the vitelline veins open into the sinus venosus. When the left horn of the sinus venosus disappears, the right vitelline trunk receives the anastomosis of the inferior vena cava and becomes its terminal segment (fig. 3).

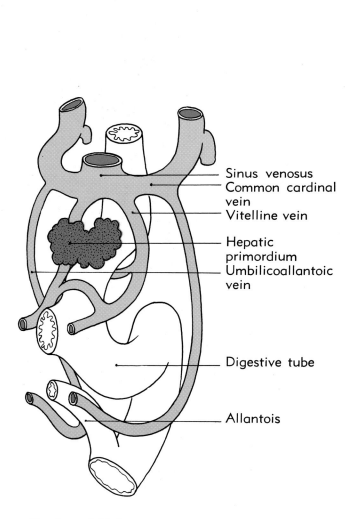

Sinus venosus
Common cardinal vein
Vitelline vein
Hepatic primordium
Umbilicoallantoic vein
Digestive tube
Allantois

Fig. 1. — *Initial arrangement*
(see p. 106).

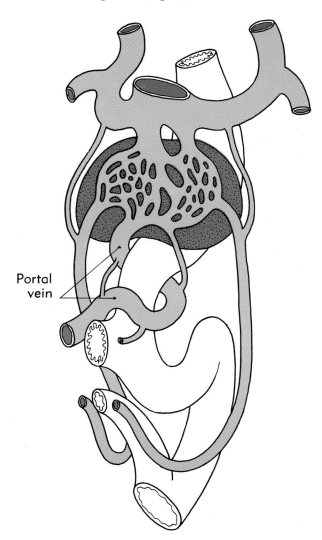

Portal vein

Fig. 2. — *Fragmentation of vitelline veins by hepatic primordium.*

PORTAL SYSTEM

The umbilicoallantoic veins, more lateral than the vitelline veins, are also fragmented by development of the liver. Their proximal portion disappears, the right umbilical vein ultimately making a complete disappearance (fig. 3).

Only the left umbilical vein continues to drain the blood coming from the placenta into the liver.

Temporarily, a short circuit is established between the left umbilical vein and the inferior vena cava. This is the *ductus venosus* (fig. 4).

The ductus venosus and the left umbilical vein are obliterated after birth.

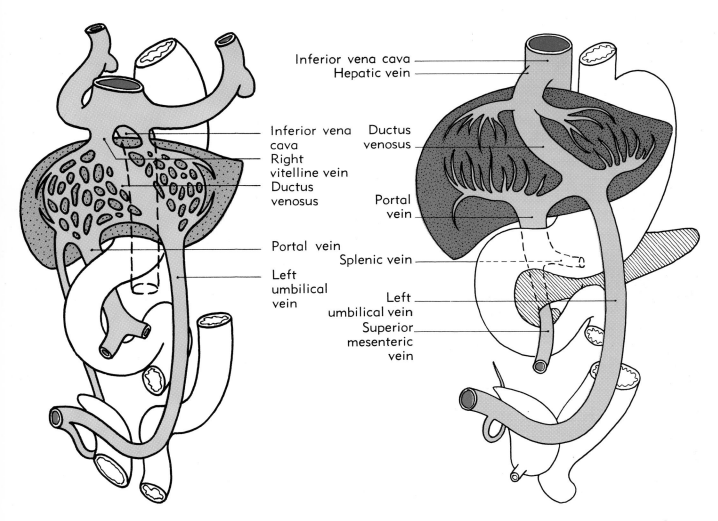

Inferior vena cava
Hepatic vein

Inferior vena cava
Right vitelline vein
Ductus venosus

Ductus venosus

Portal vein

Portal vein

Splenic vein

Left umbilical vein

Left umbilical vein
Superior mesenteric vein

Fig. 3. — *Fragmentation of umbilical veins by hepatic primordium.*

Fig. 4. — *Arrangement before birth.*

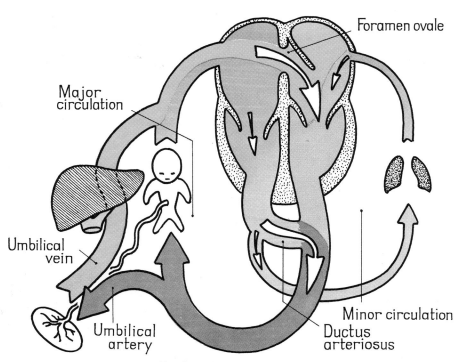

Fig. 1. — *Circulation of the fetus.*

The placenta, in addition to its nutritional role, insures oxygenation of the fetal blood. It is connected to the major circulation (see p. 120).

The fetal blood arrives in the placenta by the *umbilical arteries,* branches of the caudal aortic system. It is returned by the umbilical vein to the liver, then by the *ductus venosus* in the inferior vena cava system. The minor circulation, although existing anatomically, is almost completely short-circuited by two mechanisms (fig. 1):

— **the foramen ovale** which allows blood to pass from the right to the left heart;

— **the ductus arteriosus,** which diverts blood from the pulmonary artery to the aortic system.

Since the fetus is in a liquid environment, it cannot use its pulmonary respiratory system. The lung, however, is ready to fulfill its role from the 6th month of pregnancy. It becomes effectively functional only at the time of passage to autonomous life in an air environment.

At birth, placental circulation is interrupted. The abrupt fall in intrathoracic pressure brought about by the first respiration contributes to initiation of pulmonary circulation:

— blood pressure decreases in the pulmonary artery, although its flow is increased, since it supplies a capillary network considerably enlarged by expansion of the pulmonary parenchyma;

AT BIRTH

— as a result, blood flow decreases, even reverses momentarily in the ductus arteriosus: its muscular wall contracts and in several days closes completely;

— similarly, influx of pulmonary blood in the left atrium increases pressure, causing the septum primum to be pressed against the septum secundum, and closing the foramen ovale (fig. 2).

At this time, the circulatory system has acquired its adult form, with separation of the minor and the major circulations. However, occlusion of the two short-circuits is for some time only physiological. It becomes anatomical after several weeks by:

— fibrous degeneration of the ductus arteriosus forms the *ligamentum arteriosum* from the left pulmonary artery to the concave inferior face of the aortic arch;

— complete fusion of the septum primum to the septum secundum forming the definitive interauricular septum. Traces of the former passage, the foramen ovale, may be seen (fig. 3).

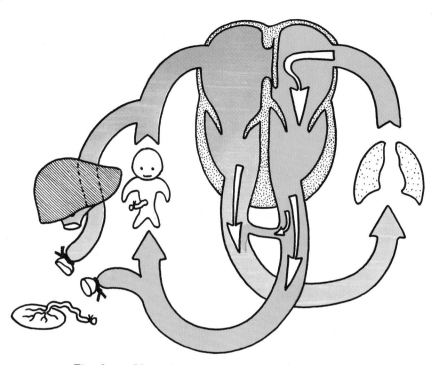

Fig. 2. — *Physiological separation of the circulations.*

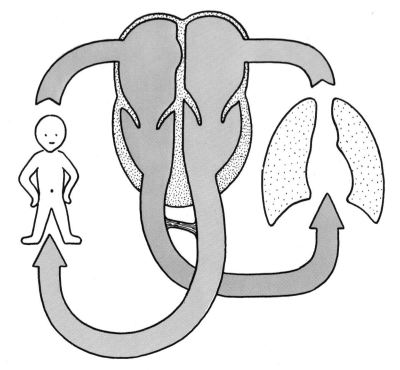

Fig. 3. — *Anatomical separation of the circulations.*

MALFORMATIONS OF THE HEART

Malformations of the heart and the great vessels are very frequent. Recent progress in neonatal cardiology permits them to be diagnosed more and more easily. Their prognosis has been considerably ameliorated by modern treatment and some are now operable.

On this page is shown an embryological classification of several simple malformations. The following page gives examples of unfortunately frequently occurring complex syndromes. The blue background in some diagrams signifies those cardiopathies which cause cyanosis. Actually, all of them are more or less cyanogenic when they reach the stage of decompensation.

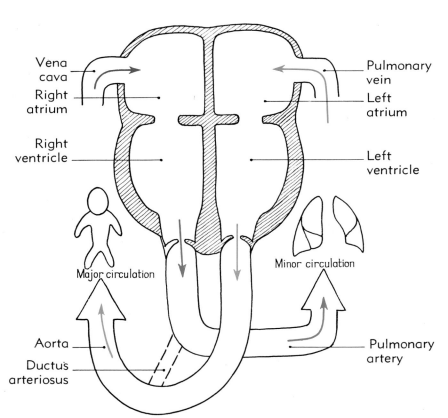

Fig. 1. — *Normal circulation.*

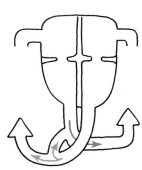

Patent ductus arteriosus.

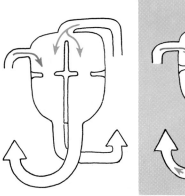
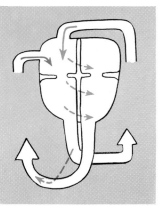

Partial anomalous pulmonary venous return.

Total anomalous pulmonary venous return (obligatory shunt below).

Fig. 2. — *Venous anomalies.*

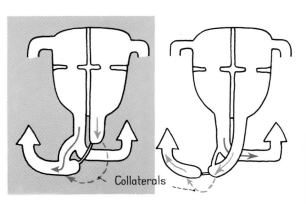

Preductal coarctation of the aorta.

Postductal coarctation of the aorta.

Fig. 3. — *Arterial anomalies* (not including arch abnormalities).

AND THE GREAT VESSELS

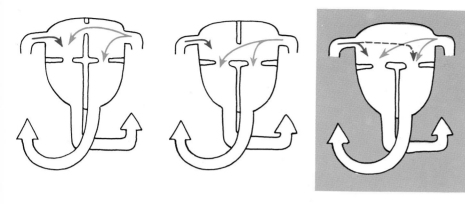

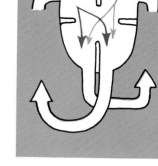

Ostium secundum.　　Ostium primum.　　Single atrium.　　Atrioventricular canal.

Fig. 4. — *Anomalies of interauricular septum.*

Fig. 5. — *Anomaly of septum intermedium.*

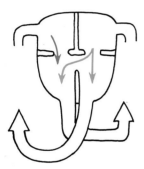

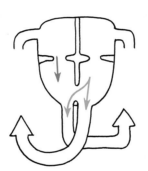

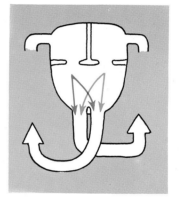

Interventricular communication, high, membranous.

Interventricular communication, low, muscular.

Single ventricle.

Fig. 6. — *Anomalies of interventricular septum.*

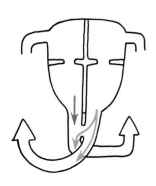

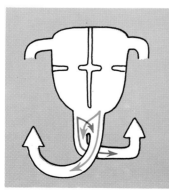

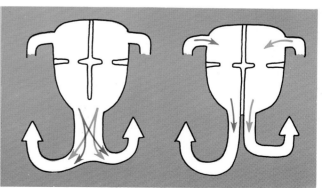

Aortopulmonary fistula.

Incomplete truncus septum.

Truncus communis.

Transposition of great vessels (preductal and postductal obligatory shunt).

Fig. 7. — *Anomalies of septation of bulbus cordis.*

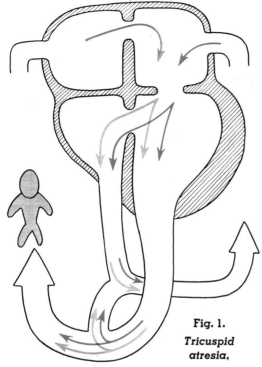

Fig. 1.
Tricuspid atresia,

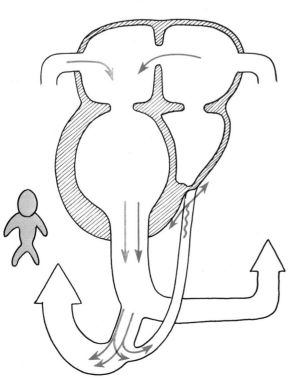

Fig. 2. — *Aortic atresia.*

Cardiac malformations often involve several anatomical defects.

Tricuspid atresia.
(absence of right auriculoventricular orifice).

This causes:

— atrophy of the right ventricle;
— hypertrophy of the left ventricle;
— intense cyanosis.

This anomaly permits survival only if it is associated with:

— interauricular communication;
— interventricular communication or patent ductus arteriosus.

Aortic atresia.
(absence of aortic orifice).

This anomaly causes:

— atrophy of the left ventricle;
— hypertrophy of the right ventricle;
— intense cyanosis.

(The coronary arteries which irrigate the heart are perfused by the aorta.)

This anomaly permits survival only if it is associated with:

— an interauricular communication;
— an interventricular communication or patent ductus arteriosus.

MALFORMATIONS

Surgical treatment of cardiac malformations does not always correct the anatomical lesion. Sometimes the methods available are only palliative and attempt to improve oxygenation. The Taussig-Blalock operation is such an example (fig. 1).

Trilogy of Fallot.

This anomaly involves:
— pulmonary stenosis **1**;
— interauricular communication **2**;
— hypertrophy of right ventricle **3**.

It causes:
— primarily: severe dyspnea;
— secondarily : often moderate cyanosis.

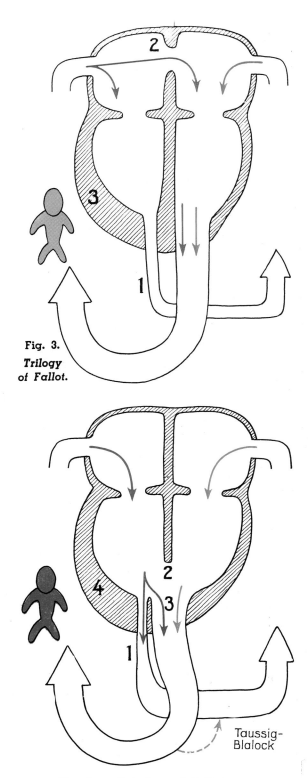

Fig. 3.
*Trilogy
of Fallot.*

Tetralogy of Fallot.

This anomaly involves:
— pulmonary stenosis **1**;
— interventricular communication **2**;
— overriding aorta **3**;
— hypertrophy of right ventricle **4**.

It causes intense cyanosis and a variable dyspnea which explains the tendency of these children to assume a crouching position.

Taussig-
Blalock

Fig. 4. — *Tetralogy of Fallot.*

SKIN AND INTEGUMENTARY STRUCTURES

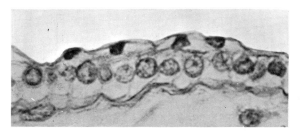

**Fig. 1. — *Embryonic ectoderm,
about 50 days* (× 77.5).**

The embryonic ectoderm (fig. 1) begins to differentiate about the 2nd month and gives rise to the *periderm*, then to the *epiderm* in two layers. Hair follicles appear about the 3rd month (fig. 2). After this stage melanoblasts, responsible for pigmentation of the skin, come in from the neural crest.

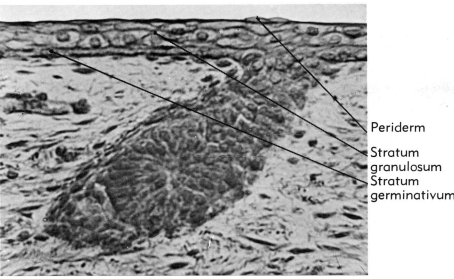

Periderm

Stratum
granulosum
Stratum
germinativum

Fig. 2. — *Fetal epidermis, about 90 days* (× 525).

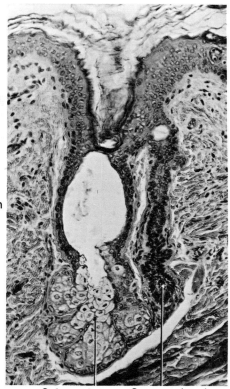

Sebaceous   Sweat gland
gland

**Fig. 4. — *Fetal epidermis,
about 8 months* (× 170).**

During the 5th month the skin completes its development into 4 layers. These layers are: the *stratum germinativum*, *stratum granulosum*, *stratum lucidum*, and *stratum corneum*. The *sweat glands* and *pilosebaceous glands* are also developped. Continuous desquamation of the cornified layer and sebaceous secretion forms the *vernix caseosa* which covers the skin of the newborn.

Pilosebaceous gland

Fig. 3. — *Fetal epidermis about 5 months* (× 180).

DERIVATIVES

MAMMARY GLANDS

The mammary glands are derived from two **primitive mammary ridges** (fig. 5), epidermal thickenings visible in the 7th week, which rapidly regress except in the thorax. The remaining mammary bud penetrates the underlying mesenchyme (fig. 6). These cellular cords canalize during the 8th month. These *lactiferous ducts* open into an epithelial depression which is transformed into the nipple after birth.

If regression of the mammary line is incomplete, supernumerary nipples (polythelia), or even complete supernumerary mammary glands (polymastia), are formed. Absence of a mammary gland (amastia) is rare.

In the newborn, mammary congestion may be accompanied by secretion of colostrum. It is attributed to transplacental passage of maternal hormones.

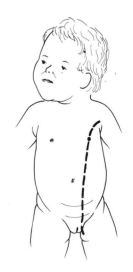

Fig. 5.
The mammary ridge.

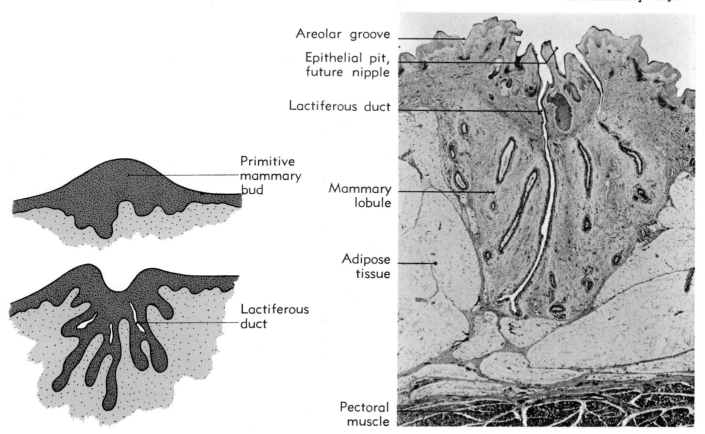

Fig. 6. — *Development of mammary primordium.*

Fig. 7. — *Mammary gland.*
Fetus of 8 months (× 20).

In the 6th week, a layer of surface ectoderm penetrates the maxillary buds. Outside this *labial groove* is the *labial lamina,* the primordium of the lips. From its deeper face, the *dental lamina* is formed (fig. 1 and 2). This plate rapidly breaks up into a number of dental buds (fig. 3 and 4).

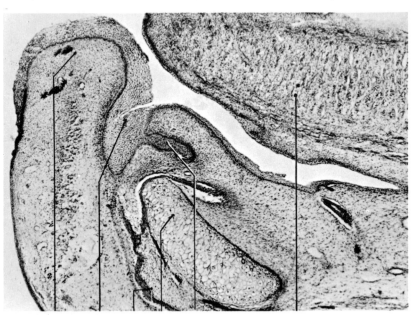

| Labial | Labial | Lower | Meckel's | Dental lamina | Tongue |
| lamina | groove | jaw | cartilage | | |

Fig. 1. — *The primitive dental lamina.*
Sagittal section of lower jaw (× 60). Fetus of 2 months.

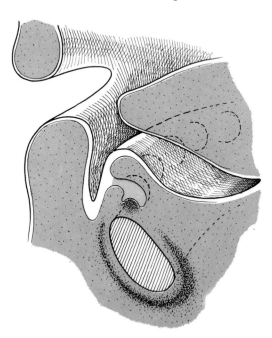

Fig. 2. — *Arrangement of dental lamina in the oral cavity.*

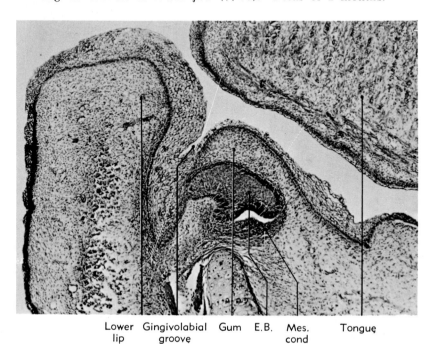

| Lower | Gingivolabial | Gum | E.B. | Mes. | Tongue |
| lip | groove | | | cond | |

Fig. 4. — *Arrangement of dental buds.*

Fig. 3. — *Fragmentation of the dental lamina : the dental buds.* Sagittal section of the lower jaw (× 70). Fetus of 2 1/4 months. (*E.B.:* epithelial bud priming a dental bell; *Mes. cond.:* mesenchymal condensation).

OF THE TEETH

Opposite each dental bud (of ectodermal origin) there is a small area of mesenchymal condensation. The dental primordium, with its double origin, is thus formed. The ectodermal primordium is organized into a *bell-shaped tooth bud* enclosing the mesenchymal primordium, the future *dental pulp*.

The bell-shaped tooth bud is attached to the gum by the *dental pedicle,* which is also attached to the permanent tooth bud.

The bulk of the bell forms the stellate reticulum.

The deep layer differentiates into a sheet of *ameloblasts.*

Opposite the ameloblasts, the mesenchyme of the pulp differentiates into *odontoblasts.*

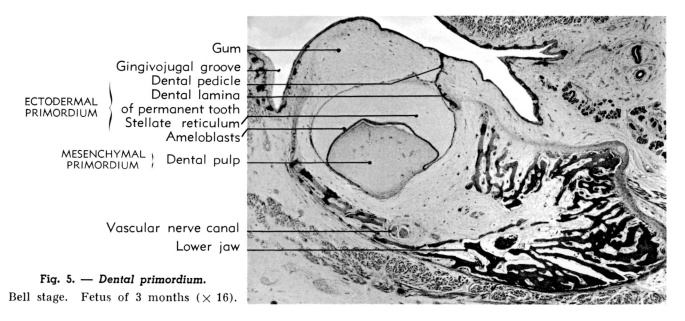

ECTODERMAL PRIMORDIUM
- Gum
- Gingivojugal groove
- Dental pedicle
- Dental lamina of permanent tooth
- Stellate reticulum
- Ameloblasts

MESENCHYMAL PRIMORDIUM
- Dental pulp

Vascular nerve canal
Lower jaw

Fig. 5. — Dental primordium.
Bell stage. Fetus of 3 months (× 16).

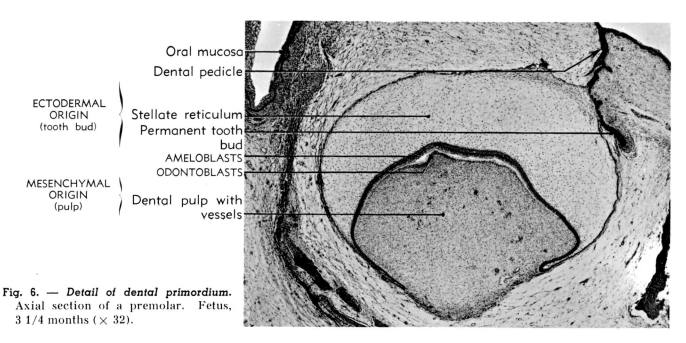

Oral mucosa
Dental pedicle

ECTODERMAL ORIGIN (tooth bud)
- Stellate reticulum
- Permanent tooth bud
- AMELOBLASTS
- ODONTOBLASTS

MESENCHYMAL ORIGIN (pulp)
- Dental pulp with vessels

Fig. 6. — Detail of dental primordium.
Axial section of a premolar. Fetus, 3 1/4 months (× 32).

DEFINITIVE ARCHITECTURE

Around the 4th month, the odontoblasts begin to secrete *predentine,* which is later transformed into *dentine.*

The ameloblasts later secrete the pre-enamel substance. These two secretions are juxtaposed in a contact layer known as the *enamel dentine junction.*

The double secretion extends over the entire face of the bell-shaped tooth bud and forms the crown, the portion of the tooth which emerges from the gum.

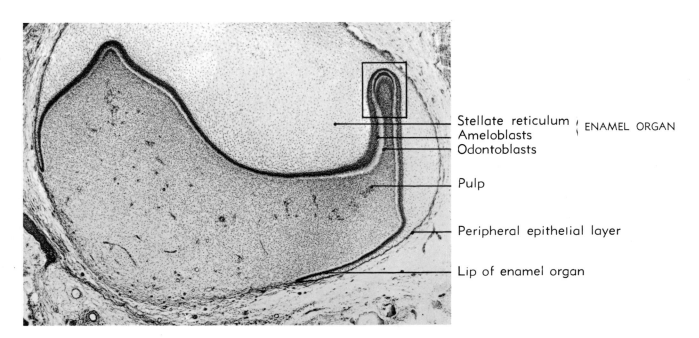

Stellate reticulum (ENAMEL ORGAN
Ameloblasts
Odontoblasts

Pulp

Peripheral epithelial layer

Lip of enamel organ

Fig. 1. — Human premolar at 4th month (× 35).

During growth of the tooth towards the surface, the stellate reticulum disappears.

The crown emerges as a nucleus of dentine covered by a layer of enamel.

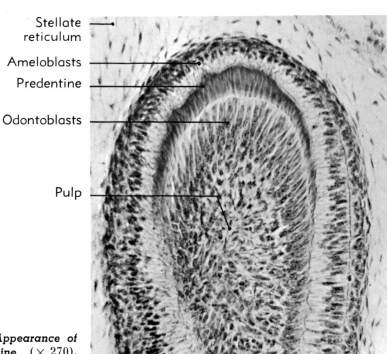

Stellate reticulum

Ameloblasts
Predentine

Odontoblasts

Pulp

Fig. 2. — Appearance of future dentine (× 270).

OF THE TOOTH

When the crown is formed, the *root* begins to develop. The ring forming the end of the epithelial cul-de-sac begins to be active.

Formation of the dentine occurs progressively with eruption of the tooth from this epithelial sheath which retracts concentrically.

Finally, about the 6th month post-natal, the tooth emerges from the gum across the vestiges of the enamel organ.

The permanent tooth buds become active about the 6th year of age.

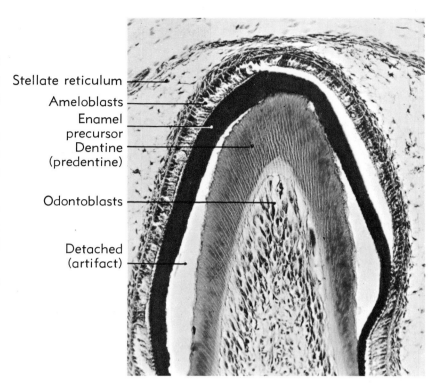

Stellate reticulum
Ameloblasts
Enamel precursor
Dentine (predentine)
Odontoblasts
Detached (artifact)

Fig. 3. — *Appearance of enamel precursor* ($\times$ 170).

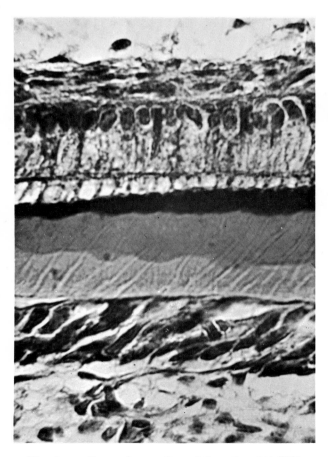

Fig. 4. — *Area of secretion elaboration* ($\times$ 700).

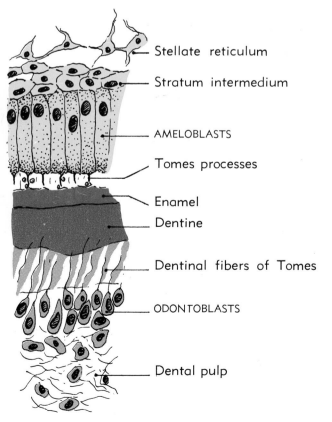

Stellate reticulum
Stratum intermedium
AMELOBLASTS
Tomes processes
Enamel
Dentine
Dentinal fibers of Tomes
ODONTOBLASTS
Dental pulp

The salivary glands develop from invagination of the surface ectoderm in the wall of the stomodeum:

— *the submaxillary bud* in the 6th week;

— *the sublingual bud* in the 8th week. Both buds develop in the gingivolingual groove, the first laterally, the second ventrally;

— *the parotid bud* in the 8th week, in the posterior portion of the superior gingivojugal pouch.

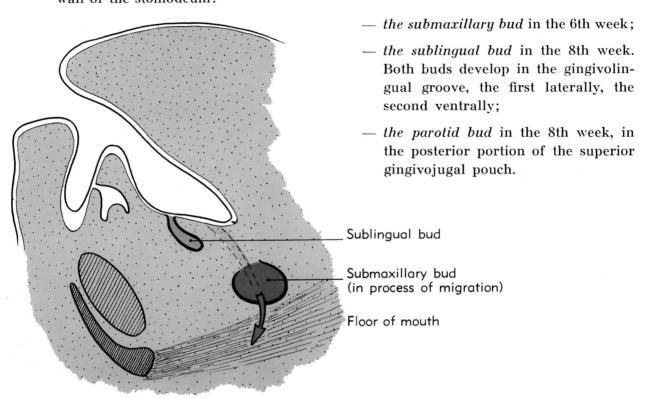

Sublingual bud

Submaxillary bud (in process of migration)

Floor of mouth

Fig. 1. — *Salivary primordia.* Sagittal section of oral cavity. Simultaneous appearance of salivary and dental buds can be seen.

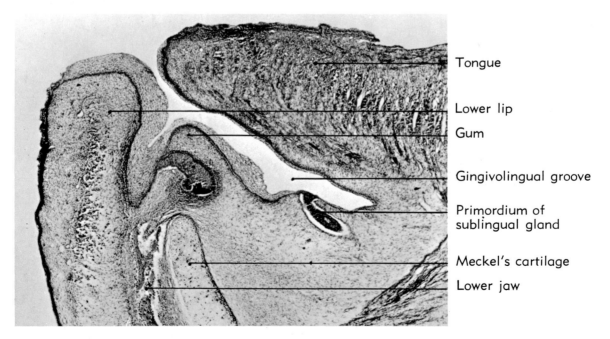

Tongue

Lower lip

Gum

Gingivolingual groove

Primordium of sublingual gland

Meckel's cartilage

Lower jaw

Fig. 2. — *Primordium of sublingual gland.* Human embryo of 53 days. Median sagittal section of the lower jaw (× 50).

THE SALIVARY GLANDS

The primitive buds penetrate the subjacent mesenchyme and divide into cellular cords, which hollow to become the first excretory ducts. The following are formed successively:

— the principal excretory duct: *Stensen's duct* for the parotid,
: *Wharton's duct* for the submaxillary;
— the interlobular ducts;
— the intralobular ducts.

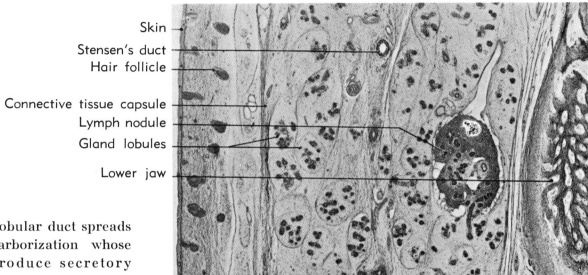

Skin
Stensen's duct
Hair follicle

Connective tissue capsule
Lymph nodule
Gland lobules

Lower jaw

Fig. 3. — *Lobular organization of a salivary gland.*
Human fetus of 90 days. Section of parotid region (× 25).

Each intralobular duct spreads out in an arborization whose ends later produce secretory acini.

The branching is contained within lobules, the portions of the gland subdivided by differentiated mesenchyme and receiving vessels and nerves.

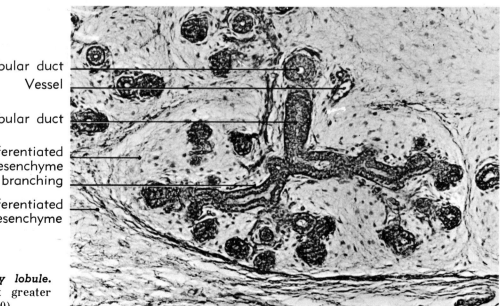

Interlobular duct
Vessel

Intralobular duct

Differentiated
intralobular mesenchyme
Intralobular branching

Undifferentiated
interlobular mesenchyme

Fig. 4. — *Salivary lobule.*
Same section at greater enlargement (× 130).

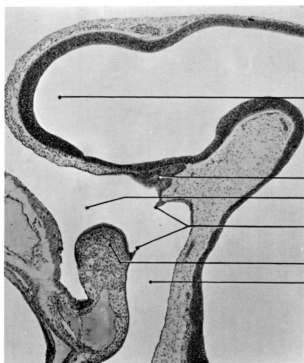

The hypophysis consists of four lobes:

— an anterior lobe,

— a middle or intermediary lobe,

— a tuberal lobe (these three lobes originate from surface ectoderm) and

— a posterior lobe (of neural origin).

Telencephalon

RATHKE'S DIVERTICULUM

Stomodeum

Vestiges of buccopharyngeal membrane

First branchial arch

Foregut

Fig. 1. — *Rathke's diverticulum.* Rabbit embryo of 11 days. Sagittal section of cephalic end (× 55).

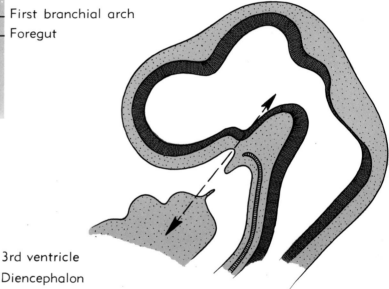

Fig. 2.

The arrow crossing the stomodeum shows the plane of section of fig. 3 opposite.

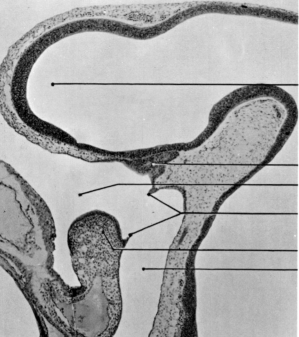

3rd ventricle

Diencephalon

RATHKE'S DIVERTICULUM

Apex of stomodeum

Tongue

Around the 21st day, a depression in the surface ectoderm in the roof of the stomodeum forms, just cranial to the pharyngeal membrane. This is *Rathke's diverticulum:* it rapidly enlarges toward the diencephalon.

Fig. 3. — *Rathke's diverticulum.* Human embryo of 34 days. Cross section of cephalic end (× 92).

ANTERIOR HYPOPHYSIS

Rathke's diverticulum quickly flattens and forms *Rathke's pouch;* it remains connected with the stomodeum by a slender attachment, the pharyngohypophyseal stalk.

About the 35th day, the diencephalon also puts forth a diverticulum, in the opposite direction, from which arises the posterior (neural) lobe.

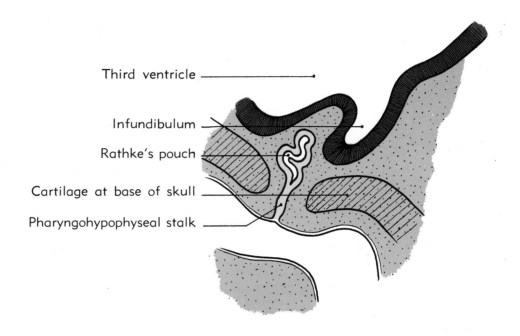

Third ventricle
Infundibulum
Rathke's pouch
Cartilage at base of skull
Pharyngohypophyseal stalk

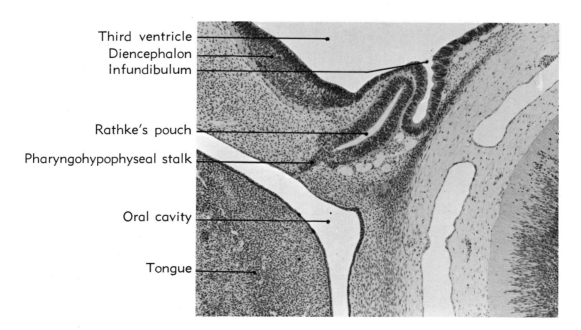

Third ventricle
Diencephalon
Infundibulum

Rathke's pouch
Pharyngohypophyseal stalk

Oral cavity

Tongue

Fig. 5. — *Rathke's pouch.* Rabbit embryo of 14 days.
Sagittal section of hypophyseal region ($\times$ 70).

Development of the cartilaginous model at the base of the skull forms a housing for the hypophysis: *the sella turcica.*

As soon as Rathke's pouch is isolated, its walls proliferate. The anterior wall gives rise to irregular cellular cords of a glandular type which form the anterior lobe.

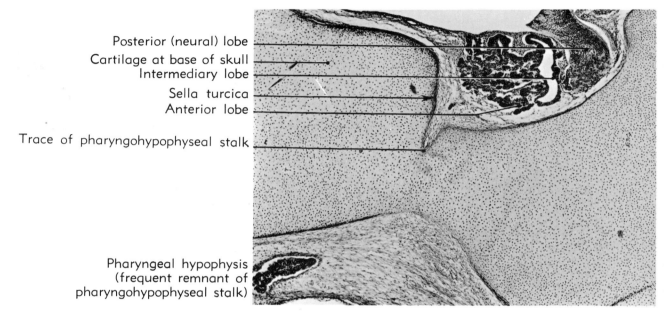

Posterior (neural) lobe
Cartilage at base of skull
Intermediary lobe
Sella turcica
Anterior lobe

Trace of pharyngohypophyseal stalk

Pharyngeal hypophysis
(frequent remnant of
pharyngohypophyseal stalk)

Fig. 1. — *The hypophysis in the sella turcica* (× 50).
Median sagittal section of base of skull.
Human fetus at 60th day.

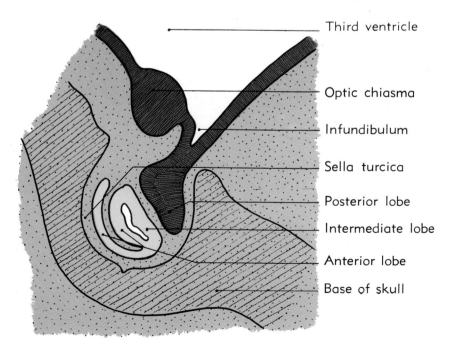

Third ventricle

Optic chiasma

Infundibulum

Sella turcica

Posterior lobe

Intermediate lobe

Anterior lobe

Base of skull

Fig. 2. — *Isolation and differentiation
of hypophysis in the sella turcica.*

Hypophyseal development is actually more complex:

— the neural lobe thickens and fills in;

— the intermediate lobe proliferates only slightly;

— the anterior lobe puts forth an extension which forms the *pars tuberalis.*

OF ANTERIOR HYPOPHYSIS

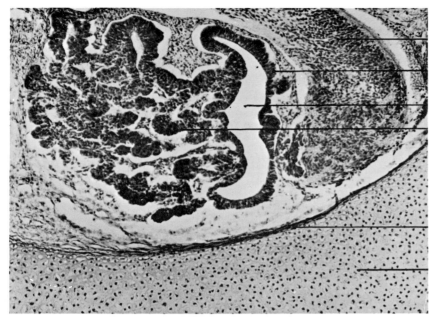

Posterior lobe, pars nervosa

Intermediate lobe

Hypophyseal cleft

Anterior lobe (glandular)
(Note selective proliferation of anterior wall of Rathke's pouch)

Sella turcica

Cartilage at base of skull

Fig. 3. — *Human fetus of 60 days.*
Sagittal section of hypophysis (× 125).

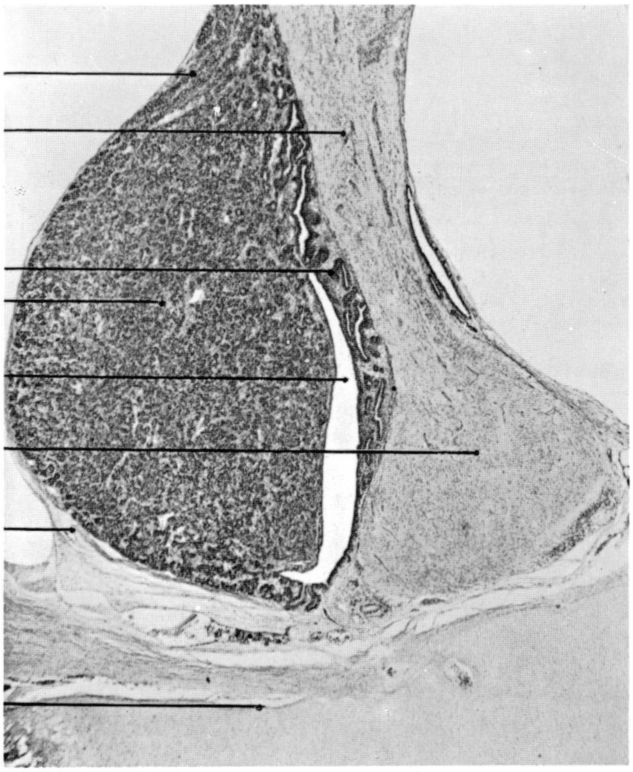

Pars tuberalis
Pituitary stalk

Intermediate lobe
Anterior lobe

Hypophyseal cleft

Posterior lobe

Spinal meninges

Sella turcica

After 3 months, certain cells accumulate eosinophil granules. Appearance of basophil granules in other cells occurs later, in the 4th month (see Volume III).

Fig. 4. — *Definitive architecture.* Human fetus of 3 months. Median sagittal section of hypophysis (× 25).

INDEX (*)

A

Allantois : **40, 66,** 72.
Alveoli, pulmonary : 47.
Ameloblasts : 141-143.
Ampulla of Vater : 35.
Androgens : **78,** 80, 82, 84, 87, 100.
Anus : 41.
—, malformations : 42, 43.
Appendix : 37.
— epididymis : 81.
— testis : 80.
Arches, aortic : 26, 122, **124, 125.**
—, branchial : 24, 25, **26.**
Atresia, aortic : 136.
—, esophageal : 49.
—, intestinal : 38.
—, rectal : 42, 43.
—, tricuspid : 136.

B

Bladder, exstrophy of : 103.
—, gall : **34,** 35.
—, urinary : 66-67.
Blastema, metanephric : 58-60, **62-63,** 68.
Bone, hyoid : **26,** 31.
Bronchi : 45, **46-47.**
Bud, tooth, bell-shaped : 141.
—, ureteric : 58, 59, **60, 61, 66.**
Bulbus cordis : 112, 116-117.

C

Caecum : 37.
Calyces, renal : 60-61.
Canal, anal : 41.
—, atrioventricular : 112-113.
—, uterovaginal : 90-91.
Cartilage, Meckel's : see Meckel's cartilage.
—, Reichert's : 26.
Cavity, pericardial : 110-111.
—, peritoneal : 32, 36, 73.

—, pleural : 46.
—, tympanic : 28.
Cells, follicular : 72, **89.**
—, Leydig : 78.
—, primordial germ : 72-73.
—, Sertoli : see Sertoli cells.
Circulation, embryonic : 120-121.
—, neonatal : 109, **133.**
—, placental : 109, 132.
—, vitelline : 104-105, 108.
Cleft, pharyngeal : 24, 25, **27.**
Clitoris : 99.
Cloaca : 40.
Coelom, intraembryonic : 2, 51.
Coloboma, facial : 20.
Column, vertebral : 4-5.
Congestion, mammary, of newborn : 139.
Connections, urogenital : 75.
Cords, cortical : 88-89.
—, medullary ovarian : 73, **88.**
—, nephrogenic : 2, **51, 52.**
—, sexual : 73, 74, **78, 88.**
—, urogenital : 57, **77,** 93-95.
Corpus cavernosum : 85, 86, 99.
— spongiosum : 85, 86.
Cortex, adrenal : 56.
Cryptorchism : 87.
Cushions, endocardial : 113.
Cysts, thyroglossal : 30.

D

Dentine : 142-143.
Dermatome : 3.
Differentiation, sexual : 100-103.
Duct, ejaculatory : **81,** 82-83.
—, Gartner's : 90.
—, lactiferous : 139.
—, Müllerian : 56, **76,** 77, 80, **90-91,** 92-95.
—, Santorini : 35.
—, vitelline : 22, **37,** 38, 105.
—, Wirsung : see Wirsung's duct.
—, Wolffian : see Wolffian duct.

* Heavy type indicates main sections.

MASSON et Cie, Éditeurs,

120, Bd St-Germain, Paris (VIe).

Dépôt légal : 3e trimestre 1982

IMPRIMERIE OBERTHUR
RENNES

Dépôt légal : 3e trim. 1982
N° 11857